Rheumatoid Arthritis

Diet Cookbook For Women

Anti-Inflammatory Recipes for Reducing Joint Pain, Enhancing Mobility, and Promoting Overall Health

KINGSLEY KLOPP

To show our appreciation for your purchase, we're delighted to offer you these special bonuses as a heartfelt thank you.

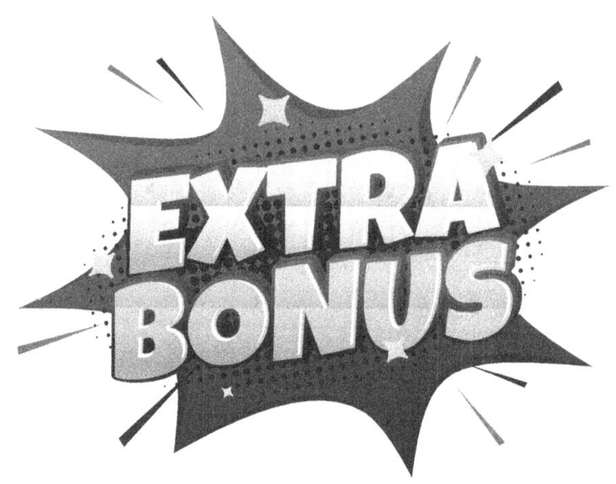

1. A Food Tracker Journal
2. Downloadable E-BOOK featuring full-color images of finished recipes

Table of Contents

Poultry Recipes

Fish and Seafood Recipes

Soup and Stew Recipes

Important Note

As you dive into these pages filled with delicious, anti-inflammatory recipes designed to help manage rheumatoid arthritis (RA), we want to take a moment to share an important message with you. Each of us is wonderfully unique, and our bodies react differently to various foods and ingredients. While the recipes in this cookbook are crafted with care to support those living with RA, it's essential to remember that what works wonderfully for one person may not have the same effect for another. Dietary needs can vary greatly from one individual to the next, influenced by factors like age, lifestyle, and specific health conditions. We encourage you to think of this cookbook as a flexible guide rather than a strict rulebook. Feel free to adjust the recipes to suit your personal taste preferences and nutritional needs. If you're allergic to certain ingredients or if something doesn't sit well with you, don't hesitate to make substitutions or skip them altogether. Your comfort and enjoyment are paramount.

Moreover, while we strive to provide accurate nutritional information, please keep in mind that these values are approximate. The exact nutritional content of a dish can vary depending on the specific ingredients you use and how you prepare them. Ingredients sourced from different regions, variations in portion sizes, and cooking methods can all influence the final nutritional profile of a meal.

We also want to remind you of the importance of consulting with your healthcare provider as you embark on this dietary journey. If you're unsure about how a certain ingredient might affect your RA or overall health, your doctor or a registered dietitian can offer personalized advice tailored to your situation. They can help you navigate any concerns and make informed decisions that align with your health goals. Navigating the world of nutrition and RA management can sometimes feel overwhelming, but you don't have to do it alone. This cookbook is here to inspire and guide you, providing a starting point for nourishing, healing meals that you can adapt to fit your life. Remember, the kitchen is a place of creativity and joy. Have fun experimenting with these recipes, and don't be afraid to make them your own. Listen to your body, trust your instincts, and seek professional guidance when needed.

Introduction

Welcome to "**Rheumatoid Arthritis Diet Cookbook For Women** , If you've picked up this book, you're likely navigating the often challenging journey of managing rheumatoid arthritis (RA). As a woman, you might already be balancing countless roles and responsibilities, and dealing with RA can feel like an overwhelming addition to your daily life. But here's the good news: you're not alone, and there's a lot we can do together to help ease your pain and improve your quality of life. Rheumatoid arthritis isn't just another health condition—it's a persistent companion that can dramatically impact your day-to-day activities. The swelling, stiffness, and pain can turn simple tasks into Herculean efforts. But amidst the plethora of medical treatments and lifestyle changes, there's a powerful tool often overlooked: the food you eat. That's right—your diet can play a crucial role in managing RA symptoms and even improving your overall health. Imagine starting your day with a delicious, warm bowl of anti-inflammatory oatmeal, sprinkled with berries and nuts that are packed with nutrients known to combat inflammation. Or picture winding down with a hearty, comforting dinner that not only tastes amazing but also helps reduce your joint pain. This isn't wishful thinking—it's a reality you can achieve with the right guidance and recipes. This book is more than just a collection of recipes. It's a holistic guide designed specifically for women who are facing the unique challenges of rheumatoid arthritis. We'll explore how the foods you choose can impact your inflammation levels, provide sustained energy, and support your body's natural healing processes. Whether you're new to managing RA or looking for fresh, effective ways to support your health, this cookbook is your companion on the journey to feeling better.

Why focus on women? Well, rheumatoid arthritis often affects women differently than men, with hormonal fluctuations and other gender-specific factors playing a significant role in how the disease manifests and progresses. As women, we have unique nutritional needs that can profoundly influence our health outcomes. This book is tailored to those needs, offering recipes and dietary strategies that address the specific challenges women with RA face. We understand that life with RA is a rollercoaster, full of ups and downs. That's why the recipes in this cookbook are not just healthy and anti-inflammatory—they're also designed to be practical, easy to prepare, and most importantly, delicious. We believe that food should be a source of joy and comfort, not just fuel. Our goal is to help you discover that eating for your health doesn't mean sacrificing flavor or pleasure.

In the chapters that follow, you'll find a treasure trove of recipes ranging from vibrant salads and soothing soups to satisfying main dishes and delectable desserts. Each recipe is crafted to maximize anti-inflammatory benefits while satisfying your taste buds. You'll also find tips on meal planning, grocery shopping, and preparing meals that fit seamlessly into your busy life. But we're not stopping at recipes. This book also dives into the science behind how certain foods can help reduce inflammation and manage RA symptoms. You'll gain insights into which ingredients to embrace and which to avoid, empowering you to make informed choices every day.

So, let's embark on this journey together. Let's reclaim your kitchen as a space of healing and nourishment. With the right tools and a sprinkle of culinary creativity, you can transform your diet into a powerful ally against rheumatoid arthritis. Let's get cooking and start paving the way to a healthier, happier you!

Chapter 1

Understanding Rheumatoid Arthritis (RA)

What is Rheumatoid Arthritis?

Rheumatoid arthritis (RA) is a chronic inflammatory disorder that can have a profound impact on your life. It's more than just the occasional aches and pains; it's a relentless battle that affects not just your joints but your entire being. This disease, driven by an overactive immune system, turns your body's defenses against itself, attacking the synovium—the lining of the membranes that surround your joints. This assault leads to painful swelling, joint damage, and can even affect other organs in the body.

A Brief History of Rheumatoid Arthritis

The history of rheumatoid arthritis is as complex and intriguing as the disease itself. Though RA may seem like a modern affliction, its roots trace back through centuries. The earliest descriptions of symptoms resembling RA date back to ancient texts. However, it was not until the late 1800s that rheumatoid arthritis was distinctly identified as a separate disease.

The term "rheumatoid arthritis" was coined in 1859 by British rheumatologist Dr. Alfred Baring Garrod. Before this, people suffering from RA were often misdiagnosed with other forms of arthritis or joint diseases. Garrod's work was pioneering in recognizing the unique characteristics of RA, distinguishing it from other similar ailments.

The Evolution of Understanding RA

Over the decades, the understanding of rheumatoid arthritis has evolved dramatically. Initially, RA was thought to be solely a disease of the joints. However, medical advancements have revealed that it is, in fact, a systemic disease that can affect multiple organs including the heart, lungs, and eyes. This revelation was crucial in understanding the full scope of the disease and the necessity for comprehensive care.

The 20th century brought significant advancements in the treatment and management of RA. The introduction of disease-modifying antirheumatic drugs (DMARDs) in the 1950s marked a turning point in how RA was managed. These drugs were the first to offer hope in slowing the progression of the disease, rather than just alleviating symptoms.

The Modern Era of RA Treatment

The late 20th and early 21st centuries have seen even more groundbreaking advancements. The development of biologic response modifiers, or biologics, revolutionized RA treatment. These medications target specific components of the immune system, offering more precise and effective control of the disease. Biologics have changed the lives of many people with RA, providing significant relief and improved quality of life.

Furthermore, the role of genetics in RA has been a significant focus of research. Scientists have identified several genetic markers that increase the risk of developing RA, offering insights into potential future therapies that could one day prevent the disease altogether.

Living with Rheumatoid Arthritis

Living with rheumatoid arthritis is a journey of resilience and strength. The impact of RA extends beyond the physical symptoms; it challenges your emotional and mental well-being. Each day can be a struggle, filled with uncertainty and the need to adapt to ever-changing physical limitations. Yet, those who live with RA often display remarkable courage and determination.

Managing RA requires a holistic approach that includes medication, physical therapy, and lifestyle changes. Staying active, eating a balanced diet, and finding ways to manage stress are all critical components of living well with RA. Support from healthcare professionals, family, and friends plays a vital role in navigating this chronic illness.

The Future of RA

The future of rheumatoid arthritis holds promise. Ongoing research is continuously uncovering new insights into the disease, leading to innovative treatments and potential cures. Advances in technology and personalized medicine offer hope for more effective and individualized care.

As we look to the future, it's essential to remember that while RA can be a formidable adversary, it is not invincible. Through continued research, awareness, and support, we can make strides towards a world where RA is not just managed but ultimately conquered.

Symptoms and Causes

Symptoms of Rheumatoid Arthritis
The symptoms of rheumatoid arthritis can vary greatly among individuals, but they typically involve a combination of joint-related and systemic manifestations. Here are the primary symptoms associated with RA:

1. **Joint Pain and Swelling:**
   - Pain: One of the hallmark symptoms of RA is persistent pain in the affected joints. This pain is often described as a dull, aching sensation that can be severe and debilitating.
   - Swelling: Inflammation leads to noticeable swelling in the joints, making them appear larger than normal and often causing a warm feeling to the touch.
2. **Stiffness:**
   - Morning Stiffness: RA commonly causes stiffness in the joints, especially in the morning or after periods of inactivity. This stiffness can last for an hour or longer, making it difficult to perform daily tasks.
   - Reduced Range of Motion: The stiffness can also lead to a reduced range of motion in the affected joints, limiting the ability to move them fully.
3. **Fatigue:**
   - Chronic Fatigue: Individuals with RA often experience extreme tiredness and a lack of energy, which can be overwhelming and affect overall quality of life.
   - Malaise: This general feeling of discomfort and unease is a common systemic symptom that can be difficult to pinpoint but significantly impacts daily living.
4. **Joint Deformities:**
   - Deformities: Over time, chronic inflammation can lead to permanent joint damage and deformities. Common deformities include ulnar deviation (fingers angling away from the thumb) and swan-neck deformities (abnormal bending of the finger joints).
5. **Nodules:**
   - Rheumatoid Nodules: These are firm lumps that develop under the skin, often near the joints. They are a visible sign of RA and can vary in size.
6. **Systemic Symptoms:**
   - Fever: Low-grade fevers can accompany flare-ups of RA, indicating active inflammation.
   - Weight Loss: Unintended weight loss can occur due to chronic inflammation and the body's increased metabolic demands.

7. Other Organ Involvement:
- Lungs: RA can cause inflammation in the lungs (pleuritis) or lead to interstitial lung disease, which affects the lung tissue.
- Heart: Inflammation can affect the heart, increasing the risk of cardiovascular diseases, such as pericarditis (inflammation of the heart lining) and myocarditis (inflammation of the heart muscle).
- Eyes: RA can lead to eye conditions like dry eyes (keratoconjunctivitis sicca) or inflammation in the white part of the eye (scleritis).

Causes of Rheumatoid Arthritis

The exact cause of rheumatoid arthritis remains elusive, but it is believed to result from a combination of genetic, environmental, and hormonal factors. Understanding these causes provides insight into the complex nature of RA and helps identify potential risk factors.

1. **Genetic Factors:**
   - Family History: Having a family history of RA increases the likelihood of developing the disease. Specific genetic markers, such as HLA-DR4, have been associated with a higher risk of RA.
   - Genetic Mutations: Certain gene mutations can influence the immune system's function, making it more prone to mistakenly attacking the body's tissues.

2. **Environmental Factors:**
   - Infections: Some researchers believe that bacterial or viral infections could trigger RA by activating the immune system in genetically predisposed individuals.
   - Smoking: Cigarette smoking is a well-established risk factor for RA. It not only increases the risk of developing the disease but also exacerbates its severity.
   - Pollutants: Exposure to environmental pollutants and chemicals has been linked to an increased risk of RA, though the exact mechanisms remain unclear.

3. **Hormonal Factors:**
   - Gender: Women are more likely to develop RA than men, suggesting that hormonal factors play a role. Fluctuations in hormone levels, particularly estrogen, may influence the immune system and contribute to the development of RA.
   - Pregnancy: RA symptoms can change during pregnancy, often improving during pregnancy and flaring up postpartum. This phenomenon indicates a possible hormonal link to the disease.

- **4. Immune System Dysfunction:**
- Autoimmunity: RA is an autoimmune disorder, meaning the immune system mistakenly attacks the body's own tissues. This autoimmune response primarily targets the synovium, leading to chronic inflammation and joint damage.
- Cytokines: Cytokines are proteins that play a crucial role in cell signaling within the immune system. In RA, certain cytokines, such as tumor necrosis factor-alpha (TNF-α) and interleukin-6 (IL-6), are overproduced, driving inflammation and joint destruction.
- **5. Microbiome:**
- Gut Health: Emerging research suggests that the gut microbiome—the community of microorganisms living in the digestive tract—may influence the development and progression of RA. Imbalances in gut bacteria could potentially trigger autoimmune responses.

The Role of Diet in Managing Rheumatoid Arthritis

Rheumatoid arthritis (RA) is more than just a chronic illness; it's a daily struggle that affects every aspect of your life. Managing this condition can often feel like an overwhelming battle, but one of the most powerful tools at your disposal is something you encounter every day—your diet. What you eat plays a crucial role in managing the symptoms of RA, potentially transforming pain into relief and helping you reclaim your life.

The Power of Food

Food is not just sustenance; it's a form of medicine, especially when living with RA. The right diet can help reduce inflammation, alleviate pain, and improve your overall well-being. This connection between diet and RA is supported by a growing body of research and countless personal stories of transformation.

Anti-Inflammatory Diets: A Path to Relief

An anti-inflammatory diet is often recommended for individuals with RA. This approach focuses on foods that naturally combat inflammation, helping to ease the burden on your joints and reduce the severity of symptoms. Here's how an anti-inflammatory diet can make a difference:

1. **Omega-3 Fatty Acids:**
   - Sources: Found in fatty fish like salmon, mackerel, and sardines, as well as in flaxseeds and walnuts.
   - Benefits: Omega-3s are known for their potent anti-inflammatory properties. They help reduce the production of inflammatory cytokines and enzymes, providing relief from joint pain and stiffness.

2. **Fruits and Vegetables:**
   - Sources: Berries, cherries, spinach, kale, and broccoli are among the best choices.
   - Benefits: Rich in antioxidants and phytochemicals, these foods help neutralize free radicals and reduce inflammation. They are also packed with essential vitamins and minerals that support overall health.

3. **Whole Grains:**
   - Sources: Oats, quinoa, brown rice, and whole wheat products.
   - Benefits: Whole grains provide fiber, which can help reduce inflammation. They also help maintain a healthy weight, which is crucial for reducing stress on your joints.

4. **Healthy Fats:**
   - Sources: Olive oil, avocados, nuts, and seeds.
   - Benefits: These fats contain anti-inflammatory compounds that can help manage RA symptoms. Olive oil, in particular, contains oleocanthal, which has properties similar to nonsteroidal anti-inflammatory drugs (NSAIDs).

5. Spices and Herbs:
- Sources: Turmeric, ginger, garlic, and cinnamon.
- Benefits: Many spices have anti-inflammatory properties. Turmeric contains curcumin, a powerful anti-inflammatory compound, while ginger can help reduce pain and improve joint function.

Foods to Avoid: Reducing Inflammation by Omission

Just as certain foods can help manage RA, others can exacerbate symptoms. Avoiding these foods is equally important in your journey to better health:

1. **Processed Foods:**
   - Sources: Fast food, packaged snacks, and sugary beverages.
   - Effects: These foods often contain trans fats, refined sugars, and high levels of salt, all of which can increase inflammation and worsen RA symptoms.
2. **Red Meat and Dairy:**
   - Sources: Beef, lamb, full-fat dairy products.
   - Effects: These foods can trigger inflammation in some individuals. They contain saturated fats and advanced glycation end products (AGEs), which promote inflammation.
3. **Refined Carbohydrates:**
   - Sources: White bread, pasta, and pastries.
   - Effects: Refined carbs can spike blood sugar levels and contribute to inflammation. Opt for whole grains instead to maintain steady energy levels and reduce inflammation.
4. **Alcohol:**
   - Effects: Excessive alcohol consumption can increase inflammation and interfere with medications used to treat RA.

Personalized Nutrition: Tailoring Your Diet to Your Needs

While general guidelines are helpful, it's important to remember that everyone's body is unique. What works for one person might not work for another. Keeping a food diary can help you identify which foods trigger your symptoms and which ones provide relief. Working with a nutritionist or dietitian who specializes in RA can also help you create a personalized diet plan that meets your specific needs and preferences.

Emotional and Mental Well-being

Managing RA is not just about physical health; it's about emotional and mental well-being too. Eating a nutritious diet can improve your mood, energy levels, and overall outlook on life. When you feel better physically, it's easier to maintain a positive attitude and cope with the challenges of living with RA.

Gender Differences in Rheumatoid Arthritis

Rheumatoid arthritis (RA) is a chronic inflammatory disorder that affects people of all genders, but it manifests and progresses differently in men and women. Understanding these gender differences is crucial for tailoring treatments and providing the best possible care for those living with RA. The disparities between how RA affects men and women can be seen in terms of prevalence, disease severity, symptoms, response to treatment, and overall impact on quality of life.

Prevalence

RA is significantly more common in women than in men. Women are two to three times more likely to develop RA, and this disparity is most pronounced during the reproductive years. Hormonal differences are believed to play a significant role in this gender disparity.

1. **Hormonal Influence:**
   - Estrogen: Research suggests that estrogen may influence the immune system, possibly making women more susceptible to autoimmune diseases like RA. The fluctuations in estrogen levels during menstrual cycles, pregnancy, and menopause can affect RA symptoms and progression.
   - Pregnancy and RA: During pregnancy, many women with RA experience a remission or reduction in symptoms, likely due to hormonal changes that suppress the immune response. However, RA symptoms often flare up after childbirth when hormone levels shift again.

Disease Severity and Progression

Women generally experience more severe RA symptoms and a more rapid progression of the disease compared to men.

1. **Joint Damage:**
   - Women: Tend to have more joints affected and experience greater functional impairment earlier in the disease. They are also more likely to develop rheumatoid nodules and extra-articular manifestations.
   - Men: Although men are less likely to develop RA, those who do often have a more aggressive disease course with severe joint damage and more pronounced radiographic changes.
2. **Inflammatory Markers:**
   - Women often have higher levels of inflammatory markers, such as C-reactive protein (CRP) and erythrocyte sedimentation rate (ESR), indicating more active disease.

Symptoms and Presentation

The symptoms of RA can vary significantly between men and women, affecting their daily lives and overall health in different ways.

1. **Pain and Fatigue:**
   - Women: Report higher levels of pain and fatigue, which can severely impact their quality of life. This may be due to hormonal influences and differences in pain perception and reporting.
   - Men: While men also experience pain and fatigue, these symptoms are often less pronounced compared to women.
2. **Joint Involvement:**
   - Women: More likely to have RA symptoms in the hands, knees, and feet.
   - Men: More frequently have symptoms in the shoulders, hips, and spine.
3. **Comorbidities:**
   - Women: Often have a higher prevalence of comorbid conditions such as osteoporosis, fibromyalgia, and depression, which can complicate RA management.
   - Men: Are more prone to developing cardiovascular diseases, which can be exacerbated by the inflammatory nature of RA.

Response to Treatment

Gender differences also play a role in how individuals respond to RA treatments, which can influence treatment strategies and outcomes.

1. **Medications:**
   - Biologics and DMARDs: Women and men may respond differently to biologic drugs and disease-modifying antirheumatic drugs (DMARDs). Women are often reported to have a slower response to these treatments and may experience more side effects.
   - Steroids: Women might need higher doses of corticosteroids to achieve the same level of symptom control as men, possibly due to hormonal influences on inflammation.
2. **Adherence to Treatment:**
   - Women may have lower adherence to RA treatments due to factors such as side effects, concerns about medication during pregnancy, and the complexity of managing multiple comorbidities.

Impact on Quality of Life

RA significantly affects the quality of life, and these effects are often more profound in women due to the combination of more severe symptoms, comorbidities, and the societal roles and responsibilities they often bear.

1. Physical Function:
   - Women with RA frequently experience greater physical disability and limitations in daily activities compared to men. This can impact their ability to work, care for their families, and maintain social relationships.
2. **Psychosocial Impact:**
   - The emotional and psychological burden of RA can be more intense for women. Higher rates of depression and anxiety are reported among women with RA, linked to the chronic pain, fatigue, and disability they experience.
3. **Economic Impact:**
   - The economic burden of RA is often greater for women, as they may have to reduce their working hours or stop working altogether due to the severity of their symptoms. This can lead to financial strain and decreased access to necessary healthcare resources.

Nutritional Needs of Women with Rheumatoid Arthritis

The Importance of a Balanced Diet

A well-balanced diet is the cornerstone of managing RA, providing the necessary nutrients to support the immune system, reduce inflammation, and maintain overall health. This is particularly crucial for women, who often face additional challenges such as hormonal fluctuations, higher rates of osteoporosis, and varying nutritional requirements throughout different life stages.

Key Nutrients for Women with RA

1. **Omega-3 Fatty Acids:**
   - Sources: Fatty fish (salmon, mackerel, sardines), flaxseeds, chia seeds, walnuts, and fish oil supplements.
   - Benefits: Omega-3 fatty acids are renowned for their anti-inflammatory properties. They help reduce joint pain and stiffness by decreasing the production of inflammatory cytokines and enzymes. For women with RA, incorporating omega-3-rich foods can significantly alleviate symptoms and improve joint function.

2. **Antioxidants:**
   - Sources: Fruits (berries, cherries, oranges), vegetables (spinach, kale, bell peppers), nuts, seeds, and green tea.
   - Benefits: Antioxidants help neutralize free radicals, which are unstable molecules that can damage cells and contribute to inflammation. Vitamins C and E, beta-carotene, and selenium are particularly beneficial for reducing oxidative stress and inflammation in RA patients.

3. **Calcium and Vitamin D:**
   - Sources: Dairy products (milk, yogurt, cheese), fortified plant-based milk (almond, soy), leafy green vegetables, and sunlight exposure for vitamin D.
   - Benefits: Women with RA are at an increased risk of osteoporosis, especially those taking corticosteroids, which can decrease bone density. Adequate calcium and vitamin D intake is crucial for maintaining bone health and preventing fractures.

4. **Iron:**
   - Sources: Lean red meat, poultry, fish, lentils, beans, spinach, and fortified cereals.
   - Benefits: Anemia is common in women with RA due to chronic inflammation and medication side effects. Iron is essential for producing hemoglobin, which carries oxygen in the blood. Ensuring sufficient iron intake helps combat fatigue and improve energy levels.

5. Fiber:
  - Sources: Whole grains (oats, brown rice, quinoa), fruits, vegetables, legumes, and nuts.
  - Benefits: A high-fiber diet supports digestive health and helps reduce inflammation. Fiber can also aid in weight management, which is important for minimizing stress on the joints.

6. Folate and Vitamin B12:
  - Sources: Leafy greens, beans, citrus fruits (for folate), meat, fish, dairy products, and fortified cereals (for vitamin B12).
  - Benefits: Folate and vitamin B12 are essential for cell division and reducing homocysteine levels, which can contribute to inflammation. Women with RA, particularly those on methotrexate, may require supplementation to prevent deficiencies.

Dietary Patterns Beneficial for Women with RA

1. **Mediterranean Diet:**
   - Description: Rich in fruits, vegetables, whole grains, fish, olive oil, and nuts, with moderate consumption of dairy and red wine.
   - Benefits: This diet is high in anti-inflammatory foods and has been shown to reduce RA symptoms and improve cardiovascular health.

2. **Anti-Inflammatory Diet:**
   - Description: Focuses on foods that reduce inflammation, including omega-3-rich fish, colorful fruits and vegetables, whole grains, nuts, seeds, and healthy fats like olive oil.
   - Benefits: Helps lower inflammation and oxidative stress, alleviating joint pain and stiffness.

3. **Plant-Based Diet:**
   - Description: Emphasizes vegetables, fruits, legumes, nuts, seeds, and whole grains, with minimal animal products.
   - Benefits: Plant-based diets are rich in antioxidants and fiber, supporting overall health and reducing inflammation.

Special Considerations for Women with RA

1. **Hormonal Changes:**
   - Impact: Hormonal fluctuations during menstrual cycles, pregnancy, and menopause can affect RA symptoms. For instance, many women experience a reduction in RA symptoms during pregnancy but may face a flare-up postpartum.
   - Nutritional Needs: Ensuring adequate intake of calcium, vitamin D, and iron is vital during these times to support bone health and prevent anemia.

2. Weight Management:
   - Impact: Maintaining a healthy weight is crucial for reducing stress on joints and managing RA symptoms.
   - Nutritional Needs: A balanced diet rich in fruits, vegetables, lean proteins, and whole grains can help manage weight and reduce inflammation.

3. Comorbid Conditions:
   - Impact: Women with RA are more likely to develop conditions such as cardiovascular disease and osteoporosis.
   - Nutritional Needs: Diets low in saturated fats and high in fiber, antioxidants, and heart-healthy fats (like those found in the Mediterranean diet) can help manage these comorbid conditions.

Practical Tips for Women with RA

1. **Meal Planning:**
   - Strategy: Plan meals that incorporate anti-inflammatory foods and ensure a balanced intake of essential nutrients.
   - Benefits: Helps maintain consistency in diet, reduces reliance on processed foods, and supports overall health.

2. **Healthy Snacking:**
   - Options: Choose snacks like fruits, nuts, yogurt, and vegetables with hummus.
   - Benefits: Provides sustained energy and helps manage hunger without contributing to inflammation.

3. **Hydration:**
   - Importance: Staying well-hydrated is essential for overall health and can help reduce fatigue.
   - Suggestions: Drink plenty of water, and include hydrating foods like cucumbers, watermelon, and oranges in your diet.

4. **Cooking Techniques:**
   - Recommendations: Use healthy cooking methods such as grilling, steaming, and baking instead of frying.
   - Benefits: Helps retain nutrients in food and reduces the intake of unhealthy fats.

Chapter 2

The Basics of an Anti-Inflammatory Diet

What is an Anti-Inflammatory Diet?

An anti-inflammatory diet is more than just a set of dietary guidelines; it's a transformative approach to eating that can profoundly impact your health and well-being. For those living with chronic conditions like rheumatoid arthritis (RA), this diet offers hope, relief, and a way to take control of their health. It is a powerful tool designed to reduce inflammation, alleviate pain, and improve overall quality of life.

The Essence of Inflammation

Inflammation is a natural response of the body's immune system to injury or infection. It's a crucial part of healing. However, when inflammation becomes chronic, it can lead to various health issues, including autoimmune diseases like RA, heart disease, diabetes, and even certain cancers. Chronic inflammation is a silent adversary that slowly wreaks havoc on your body, leading to persistent pain, fatigue, and a host of other debilitating symptoms.

The Philosophy of an Anti-Inflammatory Diet

The anti-inflammatory diet is based on the idea that certain foods can either exacerbate or reduce inflammation in the body. By carefully selecting what we eat, we can help to manage and mitigate the effects of chronic inflammation. This diet emphasizes whole, unprocessed foods that are rich in nutrients, antioxidants, and healthy fats while avoiding foods that promote inflammation.

Key Components of an Anti-Inflammatory Diet

1. **Fruits and Vegetables:**
   - Sources: Berries, cherries, oranges, spinach, kale, broccoli, and sweet potatoes.
   - Benefits: Packed with vitamins, minerals, fiber, and antioxidants, fruits and vegetables help to combat oxidative stress and reduce inflammation. Their vibrant colors often indicate the presence of powerful anti-inflammatory compounds, such as flavonoids and carotenoids.

2. **Healthy Fats:**
   - Sources: Olive oil, avocados, nuts, seeds, and fatty fish like salmon, mackerel, and sardines.
   - Benefits: These fats are rich in omega-3 fatty acids and monounsaturated fats, which have been shown to reduce inflammatory markers in the body. Omega-3s, in particular, play a crucial role in reducing joint pain and stiffness in people with RA.

3. Whole Grains:

- Sources: Oats, quinoa, brown rice, whole wheat, and barley.
- Benefits: Whole grains are high in fiber, which helps to regulate blood sugar levels and reduce inflammation. They also provide essential nutrients and can promote a healthy gut microbiome, which is vital for maintaining overall health and reducing inflammation.

4. Lean Proteins:

- Sources: Fish, poultry, beans, lentils, and tofu.
- Benefits: Lean proteins provide the necessary building blocks for muscle repair and immune function without the added inflammatory effects of saturated fats found in red meat.
- **5. Spices and Herbs:**
- Sources: Turmeric, ginger, garlic, cinnamon, and green tea.
- Benefits: Many spices and herbs have potent anti-inflammatory properties. For example, turmeric contains curcumin, a powerful anti-inflammatory compound that can help reduce joint pain and inflammation.

Foods to Avoid

Equally important in an anti-inflammatory diet is the avoidance of foods that can trigger or exacerbate inflammation. These include:

1. **Processed Foods:**
   - Sources: Fast food, packaged snacks, sugary beverages, and ready-made meals.
   - Effects: These foods often contain trans fats, refined sugars, and high levels of salt, which can increase inflammation and contribute to chronic health problems.
2. **Refined Carbohydrates:**
   - Sources: White bread, pasta, pastries, and sugary cereals.
   - Effects: Refined carbs can spike blood sugar levels and promote the release of pro-inflammatory cytokines. They also lack the fiber and nutrients found in whole grains.
3. **Red and Processed Meats:**
   - Sources: Beef, lamb, sausages, bacon, and hot dogs.
   - Effects: These meats are high in saturated fats and can increase inflammation. They also contain advanced glycation end products (AGEs), which are compounds that promote inflammation when metabolized.

4. Sugary Beverages:
  - Sources: Sodas, energy drinks, and sweetened teas.
  - Effects: High sugar intake is linked to increased levels of inflammatory markers and can contribute to weight gain, which further exacerbates inflammation.

The Emotional and Physical Benefits

Adopting an anti-inflammatory diet is not just about reducing inflammation; it's about embracing a lifestyle that nourishes your body and soul. The benefits extend beyond physical health, impacting emotional and mental well-being:

1. **Pain Relief:**
   - For those with RA, reducing inflammation can mean fewer flare-ups, less pain, and greater mobility. The right diet can transform daily life from a struggle with chronic pain to a more manageable, fulfilling existence.

2. **Increased Energy Levels:**
   - Chronic inflammation often leads to fatigue. By reducing inflammation, you can experience increased energy levels, allowing you to engage more fully in the activities you love.

3. **Improved Mood and Mental Health:**
   - The nutrients in an anti-inflammatory diet support brain health and can help stabilize mood, reducing the risk of depression and anxiety that often accompany chronic illnesses.

4. **Enhanced Quality of Life:**
   - A diet rich in anti-inflammatory foods can lead to overall better health, making everyday tasks easier and more enjoyable. It empowers you to take control of your health, fostering a sense of hope and empowerment.

Key Nutrients for Managing Rheumatoid Arthritis

Omega-3 Fatty Acids
Sources: Fatty fish (salmon, mackerel, sardines), flaxseeds, chia seeds, walnuts, and fish oil supplements.
Benefits: Omega-3 fatty acids are renowned for their anti-inflammatory properties. They help reduce the production of inflammatory cytokines and enzymes that contribute to joint inflammation and pain in RA. Regular intake of omega-3s has been shown to decrease joint tenderness and stiffness, improving overall joint health.
Emotional Insight: Incorporating omega-3-rich foods into your diet can feel like a small victory in the daily battle against RA. These nutrients offer a natural way to soothe inflamed joints, providing relief and a sense of control over the condition.

Antioxidants
Sources: Fruits (berries, cherries, oranges), vegetables (spinach, kale, broccoli), nuts, seeds, and green tea.
Benefits: Antioxidants such as vitamins C and E, selenium, and beta-carotene help neutralize free radicals, which are unstable molecules that can damage cells and exacerbate inflammation. By reducing oxidative stress, antioxidants play a critical role in managing RA symptoms and protecting joint tissues from further damage.
Emotional Insight: Knowing that the vibrant colors of fruits and vegetables signify powerful antioxidants can transform your meals into vibrant, healing experiences. Each bite becomes a step towards reducing the oxidative stress that fuels your pain.

Calcium and Vitamin D
Sources: Dairy products (milk, yogurt, cheese), fortified plant-based milk (almond, soy), leafy green vegetables, and sunlight exposure for vitamin D.
Benefits: Calcium and vitamin D are essential for maintaining bone health. RA and some of its treatments, like corticosteroids, can lead to decreased bone density and an increased risk of osteoporosis. Adequate intake of calcium and vitamin D helps strengthen bones and reduce the risk of fractures.
Emotional Insight: Ensuring you get enough calcium and vitamin D is like building a fortress for your bones, offering a sense of protection and stability in the face of RA's relentless assault on your body.

Iron
Sources: Lean red meat, poultry, fish, lentils, beans, spinach, and fortified cereals.
Benefits: Chronic inflammation and certain RA medications can lead to anemia, characterized by fatigue and weakness. Iron is essential for producing hemoglobin, which carries oxygen in the blood. Adequate iron intake helps combat anemia and improves energy levels.
Emotional Insight: Boosting your iron levels can reinvigorate your life, turning the tide against the fatigue and weakness that often accompany RA. It's about reclaiming your energy and vitality.

Fiber

Sources: Whole grains (oats, brown rice, quinoa), fruits, vegetables, legumes, and nuts.

Benefits: A high-fiber diet supports digestive health and can help reduce inflammation. Fiber also aids in weight management, which is crucial for minimizing stress on the joints. Maintaining a healthy weight can significantly improve mobility and reduce pain.

Emotional Insight: Incorporating fiber into your diet is a step towards lightness and freedom. It's about easing the burden on your joints and feeling more comfortable in your own body.

Folate and Vitamin B12

Sources: Leafy greens, beans, citrus fruits (for folate), meat, fish, dairy products, and fortified cereals (for vitamin B12).

Benefits: Folate and vitamin B12 are essential for cell division and reducing homocystcinc levels, which can contribute to inflammation. Methotrexate, a common RA medication, can deplete folate levels, making supplementation necessary to prevent deficiencies and support overall health.

Emotional Insight: Ensuring adequate intake of these vitamins is like providing your body with the tools it needs to repair and thrive. It's about nurturing your body's ability to heal and renew itself.

Magnesium

Sources: Nuts, seeds, whole grains, leafy green vegetables, and legumes.

Benefits: Magnesium plays a crucial role in muscle and nerve function and helps regulate blood sugar levels and blood pressure. It also has anti-inflammatory properties that can help reduce RA symptoms.

Emotional Insight: Incorporating magnesium-rich foods into your diet can help ease muscle tension and pain, offering a sense of relief and relaxation. It's about finding moments of calm amidst the turbulence of RA.

Zinc

Sources: Meat, shellfish, legumes, seeds, nuts, dairy, and whole grains.

Benefits: Zinc is essential for immune function and has anti-inflammatory properties. Adequate zinc levels can help reduce RA symptoms and support overall immune health.

Emotional Insight: Ensuring you get enough zinc is like fortifying your body's defenses, giving you the strength to face each day with greater resilience.

Probiotics

Sources: Yogurt, kefir, sauerkraut, kimchi, miso, and other fermented foods.

Benefits: Probiotics support a healthy gut microbiome, which is increasingly recognized as playing a role in inflammation and immune function. A healthy gut can help reduce systemic inflammation and improve overall health.

Emotional Insight: Nourishing your gut with probiotics can feel like nurturing a vital part of your inner ecosystem, fostering balance and harmony in your body.

Selenium

Sources: Brazil nuts, seafood, meats, and whole grains.

Benefits: Selenium is a powerful antioxidant that helps reduce inflammation and supports immune function. Adequate selenium levels are associated with a lower risk of RA progression.

Emotional Insight: Including selenium-rich foods in your diet is like adding a protective shield, helping to fend off the inflammation that disrupts your life.

Breakfast Recipes

1. Chia Seed Pudding with Berries

Ingredients

- 1 cup unsweetened almond milk
- 1/4 cup chia seeds
- 1 tablespoon maple syrup
- 1/2 teaspoon vanilla extract
- 1/2 cup mixed berries (blueberries, raspberries, strawberries)
- 1 tablespoon sliced almonds (optional)

Instructions

1. In a medium bowl, whisk together the almond milk, chia seeds, maple syrup, and vanilla extract.
2. Cover and refrigerate for at least 4 hours, or overnight, until the mixture thickens to a pudding-like consistency.
3. Stir the pudding well to ensure there are no clumps.
4. Divide the pudding into two servings and top each with mixed berries and sliced almonds.
5. Serve chilled.

Nutrition Info (Per Serving)

- Calories: 200
- Protein: 6g
- Carbohydrates: 28g
- Fiber: 11g
- Sugars: 9g
- Fat: 8g

Servings: 2

Cooking Time: 5 minutes (plus 4 hours refrigeration)

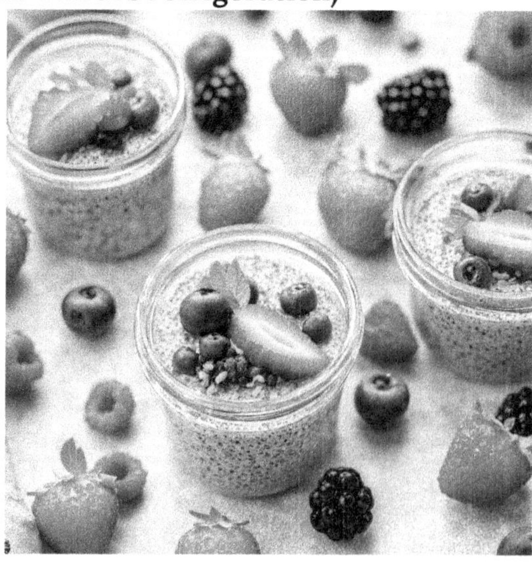

2. Turmeric and Ginger Oatmeal

Ingredients

- 1 cup rolled oats
- 2 cups water or unsweetened almond milk
- 1 teaspoon ground turmeric
- 1/2 teaspoon ground ginger
- 1 tablespoon maple syrup
- 1/2 teaspoon cinnamon
- 1/4 cup chopped walnuts
- 1/4 cup raisins

Instructions

1. In a medium saucepan, bring the water or almond milk to a boil.
2. Add the oats, turmeric, ginger, and cinnamon. Reduce the heat to medium and simmer, stirring occasionally, until the oats are tender and the mixture is thickened, about 5-7 minutes.
3. Stir in the maple syrup, walnuts, and raisins.
4. Divide the oatmeal into two bowls and serve warm.

Nutrition Info (Per Serving)

- Calories: 310
- Protein: 7g
- Carbohydrates: 55g
- Fiber: 8g
- Sugars: 18g
- Fat: 10g

Servings: 2
Cooking Time: 10 minutes

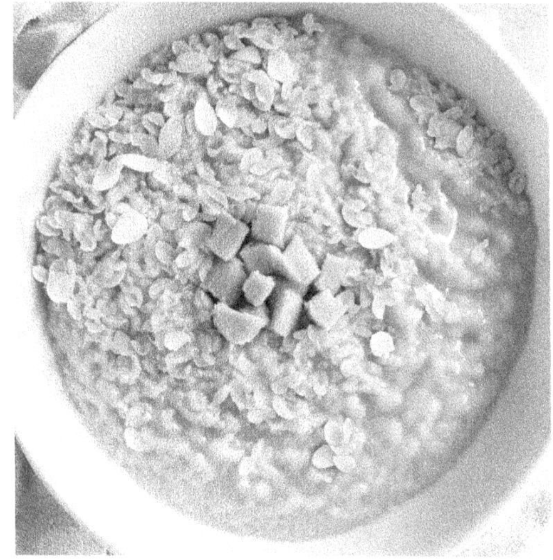

3. Smoothie Bowl with Spinach and Avocado
Ingredients

- 1 cup unsweetened almond milk
- 1 cup fresh spinach leaves
- 1/2 avocado
- 1 banana, frozen
- 1/2 cup frozen berries (strawberries, blueberries, raspberries)
- 1 tablespoon chia seeds
- 1 tablespoon almond butter
- 1 tablespoon unsweetened shredded coconut (optional)

Instructions

1. In a blender, combine the almond milk, spinach, avocado, banana, frozen berries, chia seeds, and almond butter.
2. Blend until smooth and creamy.
3. Pour the smoothie into a bowl.
4. Top with unsweetened shredded coconut, extra berries, or sliced almonds if desired.
5. Serve immediately.

Nutrition Info (Per Serving)

- Calories: 350
- Protein: 8g
- Carbohydrates: 45g
- Fiber: 14g
- Sugars: 19g
- Fat: 18g

Servings: 1
Cooking Time: 5 minutes

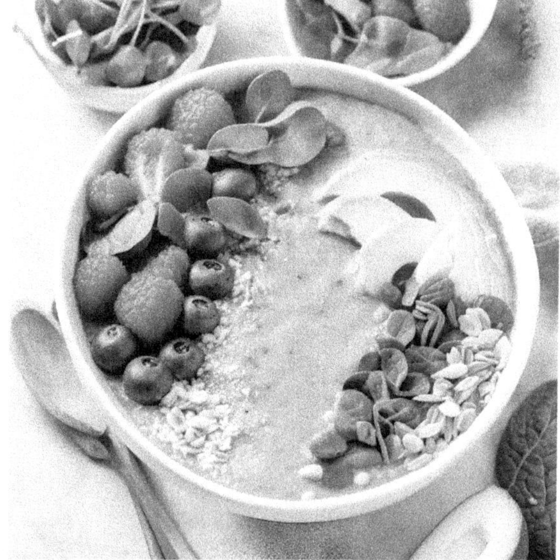

4. Gluten-Free Banana Pancakes

Ingredients

- 1 cup gluten-free oats
- 1 ripe banana
- 2 eggs
- 1/2 teaspoon baking powder
- 1/2 teaspoon cinnamon
- 1/4 cup unsweetened almond milk
- 1 teaspoon vanilla extract
- 1 tablespoon coconut oil (for cooking)
- Fresh berries and maple syrup (for serving)

Instructions

1. In a blender, combine the gluten-free oats, banana, eggs, baking powder, cinnamon, almond milk, and vanilla extract. Blend until smooth.
2. Heat a non-stick skillet over medium heat and add the coconut oil.
3. Pour about 1/4 cup of batter onto the skillet for each pancake.
4. Cook until bubbles form on the surface and the edges look set, about 2-3 minutes. Flip and cook for another 2-3 minutes until golden brown and cooked through.
5. Repeat with the remaining batter, adding more coconut oil if necessary.
6. Serve the pancakes warm with fresh berries and a drizzle of maple syrup.

Nutrition Info (Per Serving)

- Calories: 220
- Protein: 7g
- Carbohydrates: 32g
- Fiber: 4g
- Sugars: 9g
- Fat: 8g

Servings: 4 pancakes (2 servings)
Cooking Time: 15 minutes

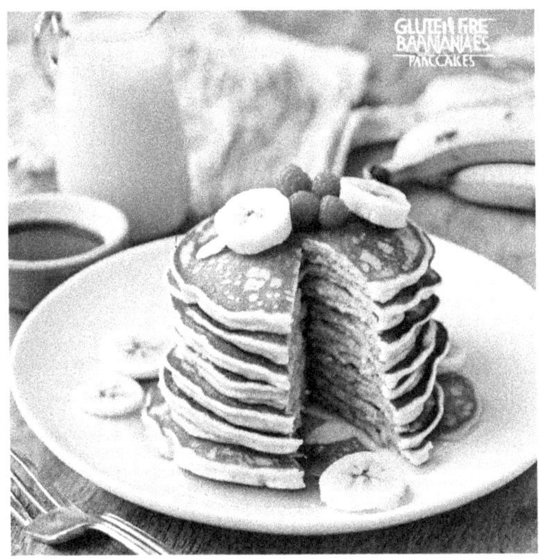

5. Buckwheat Porridge with Honey and Walnuts

Ingredients

- 1 cup buckwheat groats
- 2 cups water
- 1 cup unsweetened almond milk
- 1 tablespoon honey
- 1/2 teaspoon cinnamon
- 1/4 cup chopped walnuts
- 1/4 cup fresh berries (optional)

Instructions

1. Rinse the buckwheat groats under cold water.
2. In a medium saucepan, bring the water to a boil. Add the buckwheat groats and reduce the heat to low. Cover and simmer for 10-15 minutes, or until the water is absorbed and the buckwheat is tender.
3. Stir in the almond milk, honey, and cinnamon. Cook for an additional 5 minutes until the porridge is creamy.
4. Divide the porridge into two bowls and top with chopped walnuts and fresh berries if desired.
5. Serve warm.

Nutrition Info (Per Serving)

- Calories: 320
- Protein: 8g
- Carbohydrates: 55g
- Fiber: 8g
- Sugars: 12g
- Fat: 10g

Servings: 2

Cooking Time: 20 minutes

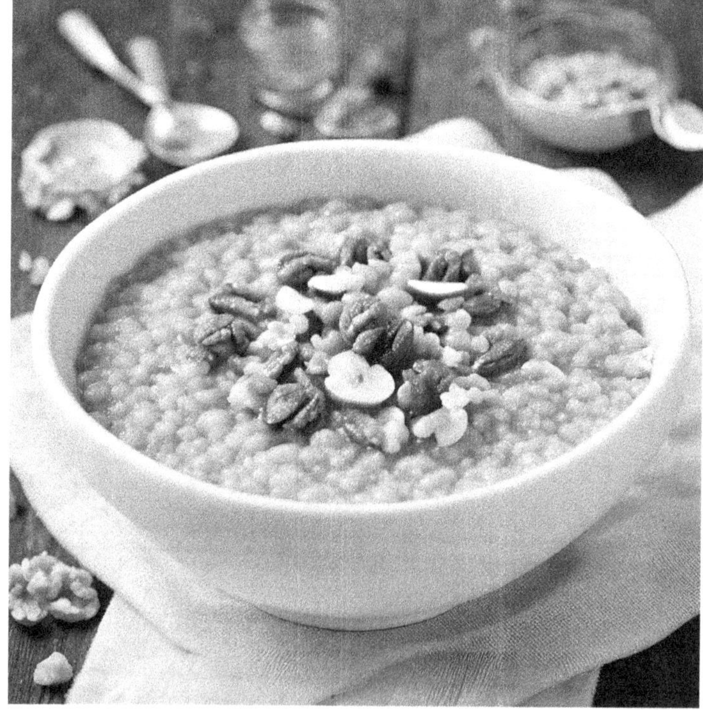

6. Baked Sweet Potato with Greek Yogurt

Ingredients

- 2 medium sweet potatoes
- 1 cup Greek yogurt
- 1 tablespoon honey
- 1/2 teaspoon ground cinnamon
- 1/4 cup chopped pecans

Instructions

1. Preheat the oven to 400°F (200°C).
2. Wash and pierce the sweet potatoes with a fork. Place them on a baking sheet and bake for 45-50 minutes, or until tender.
3. While the sweet potatoes are baking, mix the Greek yogurt, honey, and cinnamon in a small bowl.
4. Once the sweet potatoes are done, let them cool slightly, then cut them in half lengthwise.
5. Top each sweet potato half with the Greek yogurt mixture and sprinkle with chopped pecans.
6. Serve warm.

Nutrition Info (Per Serving)

- Calories: 250
- Protein: 8g
- Carbohydrates: 44g
- Fiber: 6g
- Sugars: 14g
- Fat: 6g

Servings: 2

Cooking Time: 50 minutes

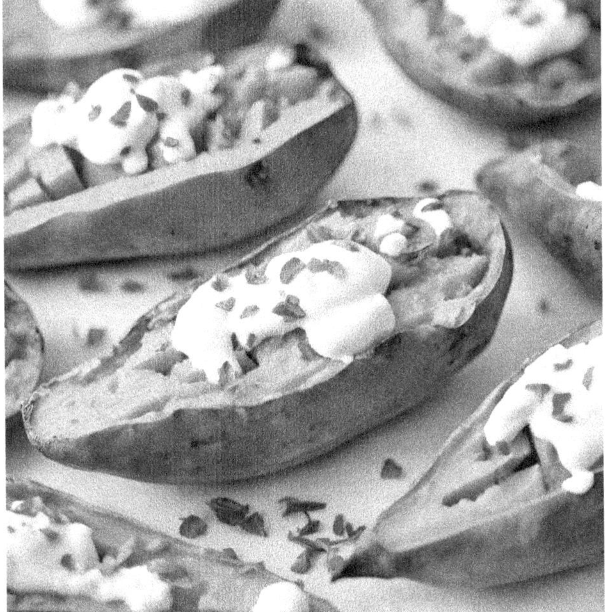

7. Savory Muffins with Zucchini and Carrot

Ingredients

- 1 cup grated zucchini
- 1 cup grated carrot
- 1/2 cup almond flour
- 1/2 cup gluten-free flour
- 1/2 teaspoon baking soda
- 1/2 teaspoon baking powder
- 1 teaspoon dried oregano
- 1 teaspoon dried basil
- 3 eggs
- 1/4 cup olive oil
- 1/4 cup unsweetened almond milk

Instructions

1. Preheat the oven to 350°F (175°C). Grease a muffin tin or line with muffin cups.
2. In a large bowl, combine the grated zucchini and carrot.
3. In another bowl, mix the almond flour, gluten-free flour, baking soda, baking powder, oregano, and basil.
4. In a separate bowl, whisk the eggs, olive oil, and almond milk until well combined.
5. Add the wet ingredients to the dry ingredients and mix until just combined.
6. Fold in the grated zucchini and carrot.
7. Spoon the batter into the prepared muffin tin, filling each cup about 3/4 full.
8. Bake for 20-25 minutes, or until a toothpick inserted into the center comes out clean.
9. Let the muffins cool slightly before serving.

Nutrition Info (Per Muffin)

- Calories: 150
- Protein: 5g
- Carbohydrates: 10g
- Fiber: 2g
- Sugars: 2g
- Fat: 10g

Servings: 12 muffins
Cooking Time: 30 minutes

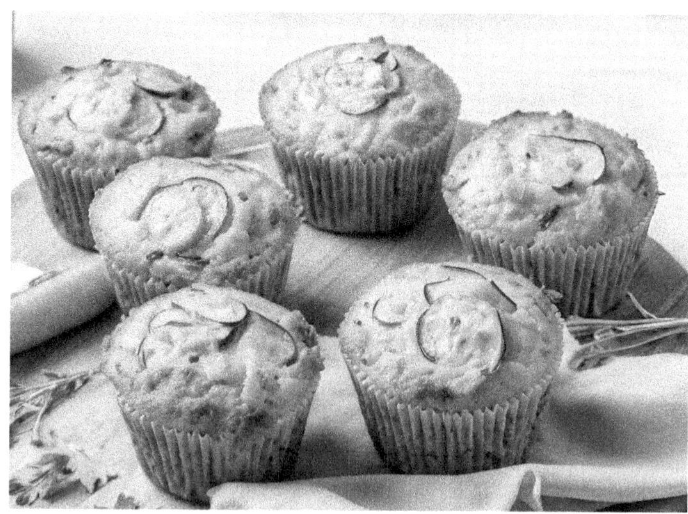

8. **Smoked Salmon and Avocado Toast on Gluten-Free Bread**

Ingredients

- 2 slices gluten-free bread
- 1 ripe avocado
- 4 ounces smoked salmon
- 1 tablespoon lemon juice
- 1 tablespoon chopped fresh dill
- 1/2 cup arugula

Instructions

1. Toast the gluten-free bread slices until golden brown.
2. In a small bowl, mash the avocado with the lemon juice.
3. Spread the mashed avocado evenly over the toasted bread.
4. Top with smoked salmon slices and sprinkle with fresh dill.
5. Add a handful of arugula on top.
6. Serve immediately.

Nutrition Info (Per Serving)

- Calories: 300
- Protein: 14g
- Carbohydrates: 26g
- Fiber: 8g
- Sugars: 2g
- Fat: 18g

Servings: 2
Cooking Time: 10 minutes

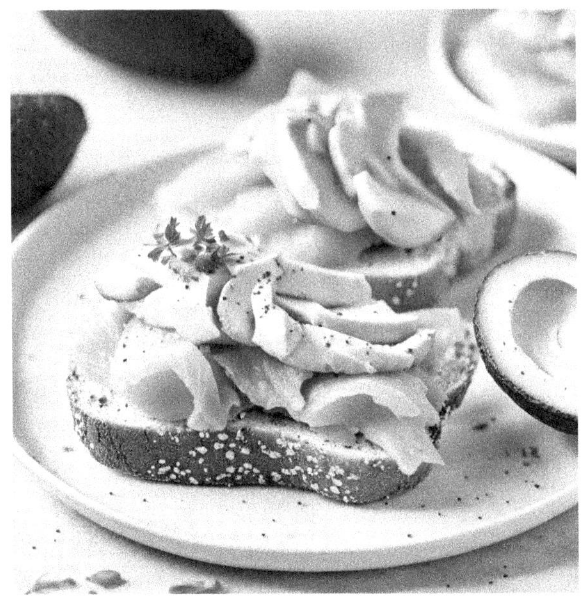

9. Almond Butter and Banana Smoothie

Ingredients

- 1 banana, frozen
- 1 tablespoon almond butter
- 1 cup unsweetened almond milk
- 1 tablespoon chia seeds
- 1/2 teaspoon vanilla extract
- 1/2 teaspoon cinnamon

Instructions

1. In a blender, combine the frozen banana, almond butter, almond milk, chia seeds, vanilla extract, and cinnamon.
2. Blend until smooth and creamy.
3. Pour into a glass and serve immediately.

Nutrition Info (Per Serving)

- Calories: 300
- Protein: 7g
- Carbohydrates: 39g
- Fiber: 9g
- Sugars: 15g
- Fat: 14g

Servings: 1
Cooking Time: 5 minutes

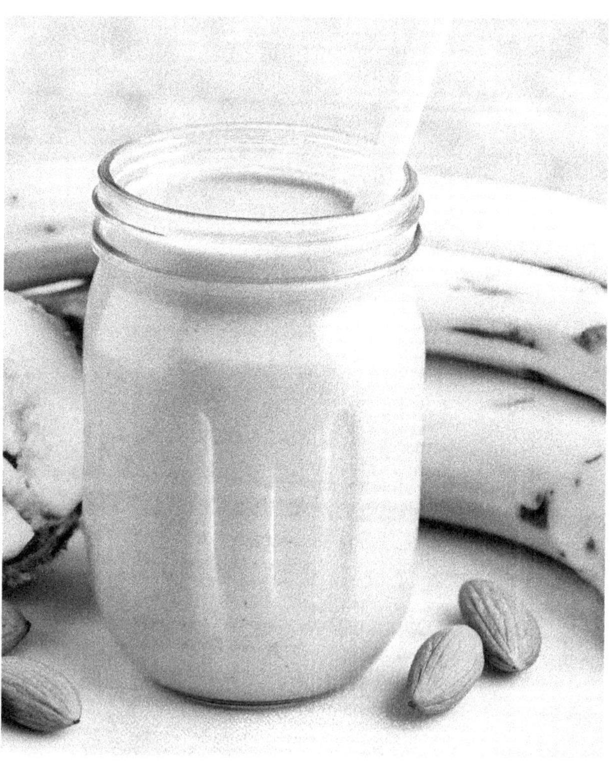

10. Quinoa Salad with Cherry Tomatoes and Kale

Ingredients

- 1 cup quinoa
- 2 cups water
- 1 cup cherry tomatoes, halved
- 2 cups kale, chopped
- 1/4 cup red onion, finely chopped
- 1/4 cup feta cheese, crumbled (optional)
- 1/4 cup chopped fresh parsley
- 2 tablespoons olive oil
- 1 tablespoon lemon juice
- 1 teaspoon dried oregano

Instructions

1. Rinse the quinoa under cold water.
2. In a medium saucepan, bring the water to a boil. Add the quinoa, reduce heat to low, cover, and simmer for 15 minutes, or until the water is absorbed and the quinoa is tender.
3. In a large bowl, combine the cooked quinoa, cherry tomatoes, kale, red onion, feta cheese (if using), and parsley.
4. In a small bowl, whisk together the olive oil, lemon juice, and oregano.
5. Pour the dressing over the salad and toss to combine.
6. Serve immediately or refrigerate for later.

Nutrition Info (Per Serving)

- Calories: 280
- Protein: 8g
- Carbohydrates: 32g
- Fiber: 5g
- Sugars: 4g
- Fat: 14g

Servings: 4
Cooking Time: 20 minutes

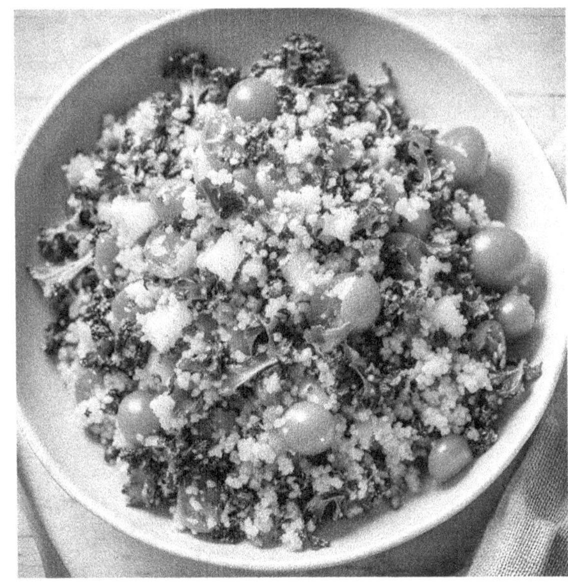

11. Stewed Pears with Cinnamon and Clove

Ingredients

- 4 ripe pears, peeled, cored, and quartered
- 2 cups water
- 1/4 cup honey
- 1 cinnamon stick
- 4 whole cloves
- 1 teaspoon vanilla extract

Instructions

1. In a medium saucepan, combine the water, honey, cinnamon stick, and cloves. Bring to a boil.
2. Add the pear quarters and reduce the heat to a simmer.
3. Cover and simmer for 15-20 minutes, or until the pears are tender.
4. Remove the pears with a slotted spoon and set aside.
5. Continue to simmer the liquid until it reduces to a syrupy consistency, about 5-10 minutes.
6. Remove the cinnamon stick and cloves, and stir in the vanilla extract.
7. Pour the syrup over the pears and serve warm or chilled.

Nutrition Info (Per Serving)

- Calories: 150
- Protein: 0.5g
- Carbohydrates: 39g
- Fiber: 6g
- Sugars: 29g
- Fat: 0g

Servings: 4
Cooking Time: 30 minutes

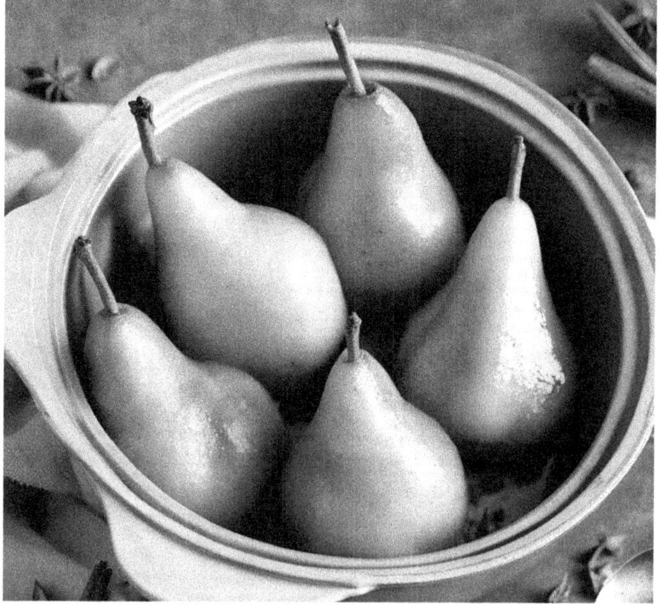

12. Kale and Blueberry Smoothie

Ingredients

- 1 cup fresh kale leaves, chopped
- 1 cup frozen blueberries
- 1 banana
- 1 cup unsweetened almond milk
- 1 tablespoon chia seeds
- 1 teaspoon honey (optional)

Instructions

1. In a blender, combine the kale, blueberries, banana, almond milk, and chia seeds.
2. Blend until smooth and creamy.
3. Taste and add honey if desired, then blend again.
4. Pour into a glass and serve immediately.

Nutrition Info (Per Serving)

- Calories: 220
- Protein: 4g
- Carbohydrates: 44g
- Fiber: 10g
- Sugars: 24g
- Fat: 5g

Servings: 1
Cooking Time: 5 minutes

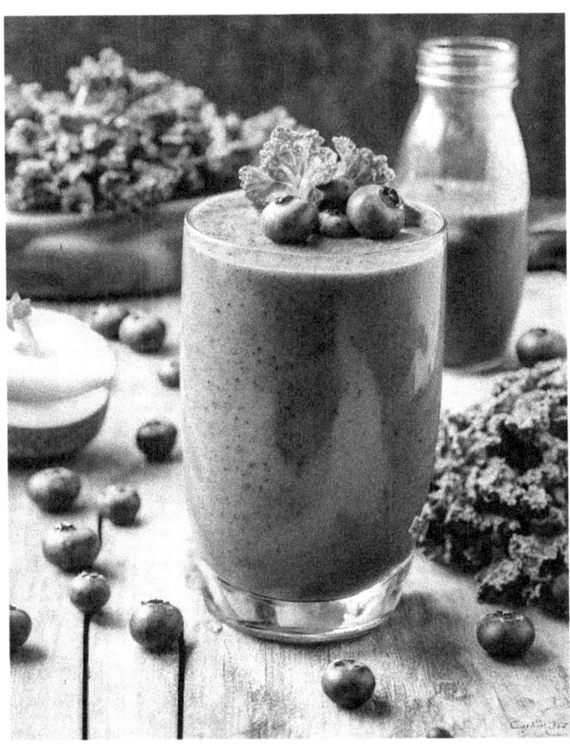

13. Gluten-Free Apple Muffins

Ingredients

- 1 cup gluten-free flour blend
- 1/2 cup almond flour
- 1 teaspoon baking powder
- 1/2 teaspoon baking soda
- 1 teaspoon cinnamon
- 1/2 teaspoon ground nutmeg
- 1/4 cup honey
- 1/4 cup unsweetened applesauce
- 1/4 cup olive oil
- 2 eggs
- 1 teaspoon vanilla extract
- 1 cup grated apple (about 1 medium apple)

Instructions

1. Preheat the oven to 350°F (175°C). Line a muffin tin with paper liners or grease with olive oil.
2. In a large bowl, whisk together the gluten-free flour, almond flour, baking powder, baking soda, cinnamon, and nutmeg.
3. In another bowl, mix the honey, applesauce, olive oil, eggs, and vanilla extract until well combined.
4. Add the wet ingredients to the dry ingredients and stir until just combined.
5. Fold in the grated apple.
6. Divide the batter evenly among the muffin cups.
7. Bake for 20-25 minutes, or until a toothpick inserted into the center of a muffin comes out clean.
8. Let the muffins cool slightly before serving.

Nutrition Info (Per Muffin)

- Calories: 180
- Protein: 4g
- Carbohydrates: 24g
- Fiber: 3g
- Sugars: 12g
- Fat: 8g

Servings: 12 muffins
Cooking Time: 30 minutes

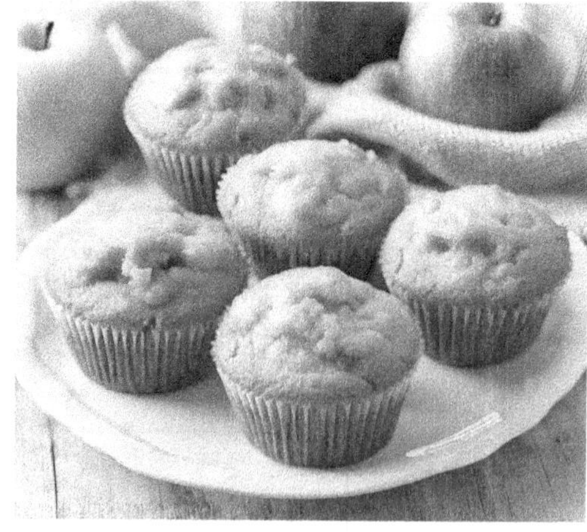

14. Greek Yogurt Parfait with Mixed Nuts and Honey

Ingredients

- 2 cups Greek yogurt
- 1/4 cup honey
- 1/2 cup mixed nuts (almonds, walnuts, pecans), chopped
- 1/2 cup fresh berries (blueberries, raspberries, strawberries)
- 1 teaspoon ground cinnamon

Instructions

1. In a medium bowl, mix the Greek yogurt and honey until well combined.
2. In four serving glasses or bowls, layer the yogurt mixture, mixed nuts, and fresh berries.
3. Sprinkle each parfait with a pinch of ground cinnamon.
4. Serve immediately or refrigerate until ready to serve.

Nutrition Info (Per Serving)

- Calories: 250
- Protein: 10g
- Carbohydrates: 30g
- Fiber: 4g
- Sugars: 20g
- Fat: 10g

Servings: 4

Cooking Time: 10 minutes

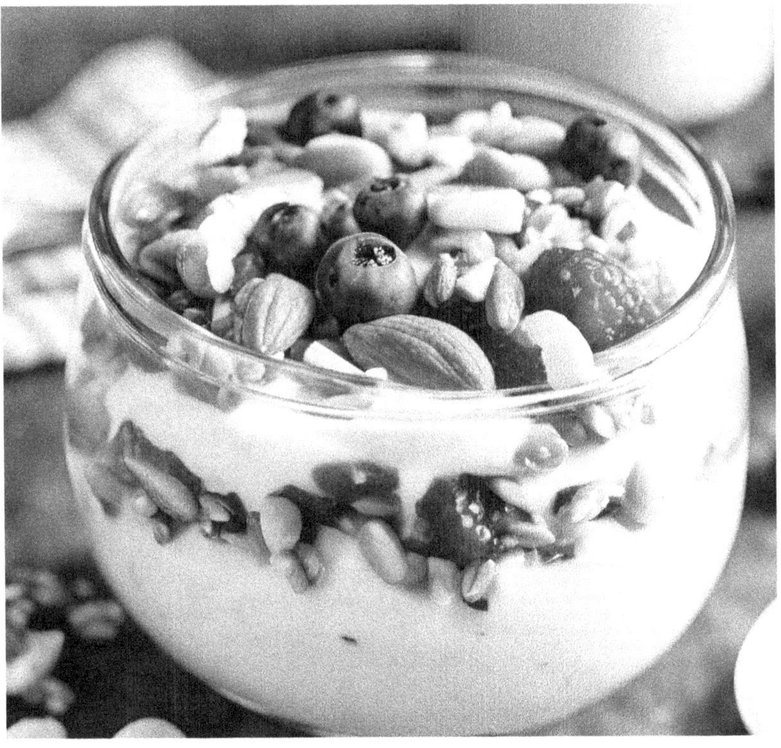

15. Ricotta and Basil Omelet

Ingredients

- 3 large eggs
- 1/4 cup ricotta cheese
- 1/4 cup fresh basil leaves, chopped
- 1 tablespoon olive oil
- 1/4 teaspoon garlic powder

Instructions

1. In a medium bowl, whisk the eggs until well combined.
2. Stir in the ricotta cheese, chopped basil, and garlic powder.
3. Heat the olive oil in a non-stick skillet over medium heat.
4. Pour the egg mixture into the skillet and cook until the edges start to set, about 2-3 minutes.
5. Gently lift the edges of the omelet with a spatula and tilt the pan to let the uncooked eggs flow underneath.
6. Cook until the omelet is set but still slightly runny in the center, about 2 minutes more.
7. Fold the omelet in half and slide onto a plate.
8. Serve warm.

Nutrition Info (Per Serving)

- Calories: 290
- Protein: 16g
- Carbohydrates: 4g
- Fiber: 1g
- Sugars: 1g
- Fat: 24g

Servings: 1
Cooking Time: 10 minutes

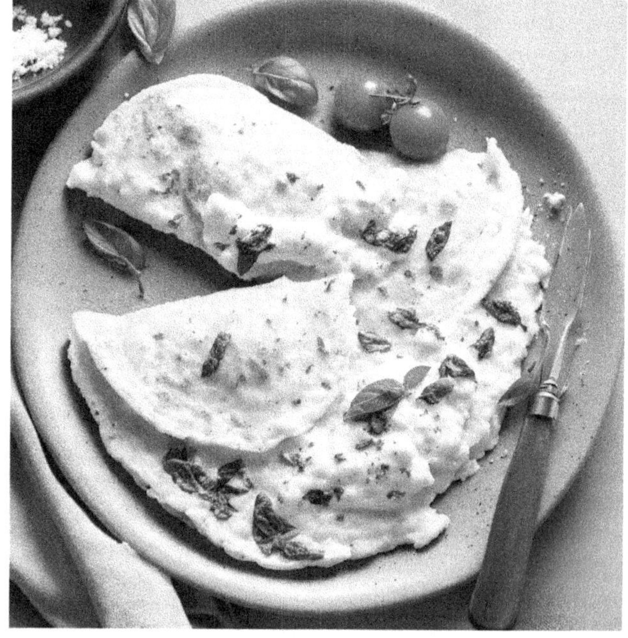

16. Pumpkin Seed Granola with Almond Milk

Ingredients

- 2 cups rolled oats (gluten-free if necessary)
- 1/2 cup pumpkin seeds
- 1/2 cup chopped almonds
- 1/4 cup sunflower seeds
- 1/4 cup honey
- 1/4 cup coconut oil, melted
- 1 teaspoon vanilla extract
- 1 teaspoon ground cinnamon
- 2 cups unsweetened almond milk

Instructions

1. Preheat the oven to 300°F (150°C). Line a baking sheet with parchment paper.
2. In a large bowl, combine the oats, pumpkin seeds, chopped almonds, and sunflower seeds.
3. In a small bowl, mix the honey, melted coconut oil, vanilla extract, and ground cinnamon.
4. Pour the honey mixture over the dry ingredients and stir until well coated.
5. Spread the mixture evenly on the prepared baking sheet.
6. Bake for 25-30 minutes, stirring halfway through, until the granola is golden brown.
7. Let the granola cool completely on the baking sheet.
8. Serve 1/2 cup of granola with 1/2 cup of almond milk per serving.

Nutrition Info (Per Serving with Almond Milk)

- Calories: 300
- Protein: 6g
- Carbohydrates: 35g
- Fiber: 6g
- Sugars: 14g
- Fat: 16g

Servings: 6

Cooking Time: 30 minutes

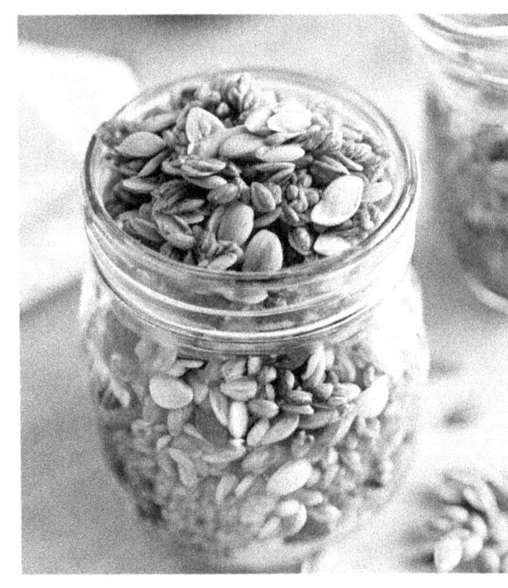

17. Avocado and Egg Breakfast Pizza on Cauliflower Crust

Ingredients

- 1 small cauliflower head, grated
- 1/4 cup grated Parmesan cheese
- 1/4 cup almond flour
- 1 large egg, beaten
- 1 teaspoon dried oregano
- 1 avocado, sliced
- 2 eggs, poached or fried
- 1/4 cup cherry tomatoes, halved
- Fresh basil leaves for garnish

Instructions

1. Preheat the oven to 400°F (200°C). Line a baking sheet with parchment paper.
2. In a large bowl, mix the grated cauliflower, Parmesan cheese, almond flour, beaten egg, and dried oregano until well combined.
3. Spread the mixture onto the prepared baking sheet, forming a pizza crust about 1/4 inch thick.
4. Bake for 20-25 minutes, or until the crust is golden brown and firm.
5. Remove the crust from the oven and let it cool slightly.
6. Top the crust with avocado slices, poached or fried eggs, and cherry tomatoes.
7. Garnish with fresh basil leaves.
8. Serve immediately.

Nutrition Info (Per Serving)

- Calories: 320
- Protein: 14g
- Carbohydrates: 15g
- Fiber: 8g
- Sugars: 3g
- Fat: 24g

Servings: 2

Cooking Time: 30 minutes

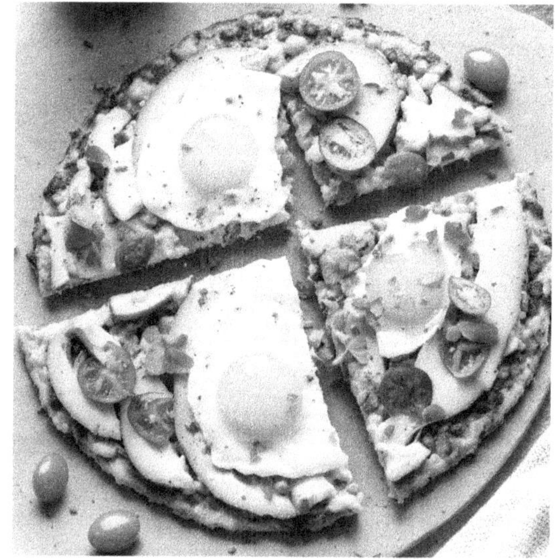

18. Berry and Yogurt Smoothie

Ingredients

- 1 cup Greek yogurt
- 1 cup frozen mixed berries (strawberries, blueberries, raspberries)
- 1 banana
- 1 tablespoon honey
- 1 cup unsweetened almond milk

Instructions

1. In a blender, combine the Greek yogurt, mixed berries, banana, honey, and almond milk.
2. Blend until smooth and creamy.
3. Pour into a glass and serve immediately.

Nutrition Info (Per Serving)

- Calories: 250
- Protein: 10g
- Carbohydrates: 40g
- Fiber: 6g
- Sugars: 30g
- Fat: 5g

Servings: 2
Cooking Time: 5 minutes

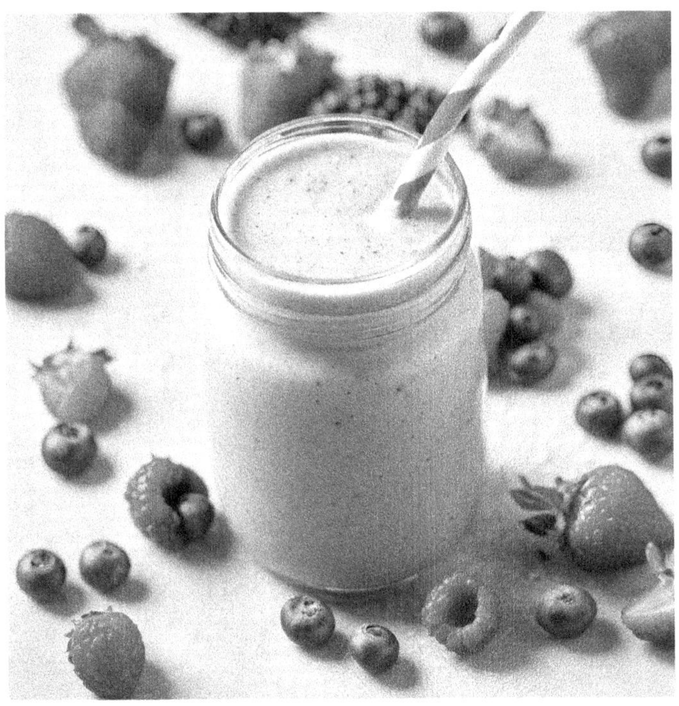

19. Sweet Potato and Black Bean Breakfast Burrito

Ingredients

- 1 large sweet potato, peeled and diced
- 1 cup canned black beans, drained and rinsed
- 1/2 teaspoon ground cumin
- 1/2 teaspoon ground paprika
- 1/4 cup chopped fresh cilantro
- 2 large gluten-free tortillas
- 1/2 avocado, sliced
- 1/4 cup salsa

Instructions

1. Steam or boil the diced sweet potato until tender, about 10-15 minutes.
2. In a medium bowl, mash the sweet potato slightly and mix with black beans, cumin, paprika, and cilantro.
3. Warm the tortillas in a dry skillet over medium heat.
4. Divide the sweet potato and black bean mixture between the two tortillas.
5. Top each with avocado slices and salsa.
6. Roll up the tortillas to form burritos.
7. Serve warm.

Nutrition Info (Per Serving)

- Calories: 350
- Protein: 10g
- Carbohydrates: 60g
- Fiber: 14g
- Sugars: 5g
- Fat: 10g

Servings: 2

Cooking Time: 20 minutes

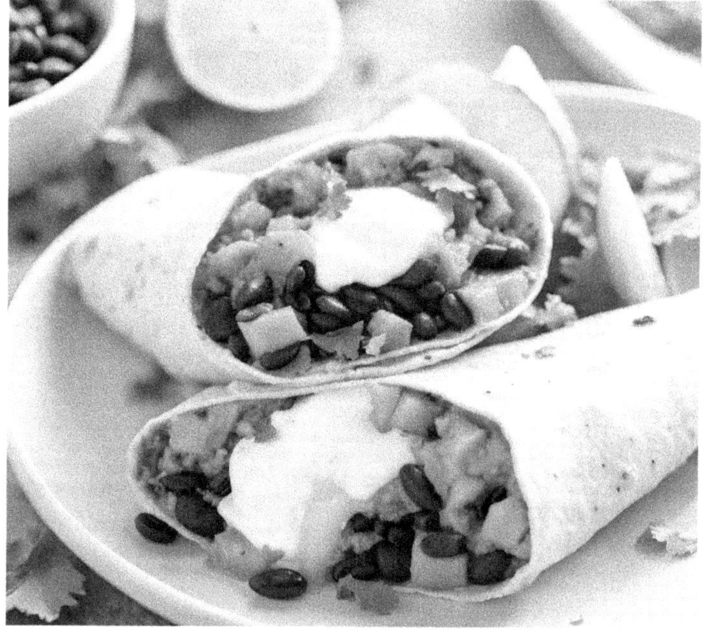

20. Millet Porridge with Apples and Nuts

Ingredients

- 1 cup millet
- 2 cups water
- 2 cups unsweetened almond milk
- 1 apple, peeled, cored, and diced
- 1 tablespoon honey
- 1 teaspoon ground cinnamon
- 1/4 cup chopped nuts (walnuts, almonds, pecans)

Instructions

1. Rinse the millet under cold water.
2. In a medium saucepan, bring the water to a boil. Add the millet, reduce heat to low, cover, and simmer for 20 minutes.
3. Stir in the almond milk, apple, honey, and cinnamon. Continue to cook, stirring occasionally, until the millet is tender and creamy, about 10 more minutes.
4. Divide the porridge into four bowls and top with chopped nuts.
5. Serve warm.

Nutrition Info (Per Serving)

- Calories: 300
- Protein: 7g
- Carbohydrates: 45g
- Fiber: 6g
- Sugars: 12g
- Fat: 10g

Servings: 4

Cooking Time: 30 minutes

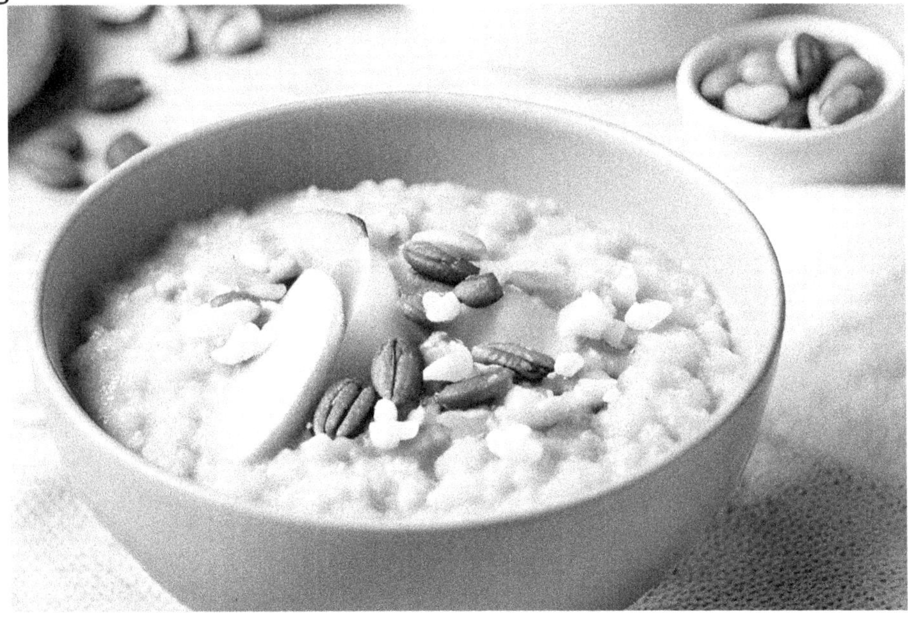

21. Cucumber and Hummus on Rice Cakes

Ingredients

- 4 rice cakes
- 1 cup hummus
- 1 cucumber, thinly sliced
- 1 tablespoon olive oil
- 1 teaspoon dried dill

Instructions

1. Spread 1/4 cup of hummus on each rice cake.
2. Arrange cucumber slices on top of the hummus.
3. Drizzle with olive oil and sprinkle with dried dill.
4. Serve immediately.

Nutrition Info (Per Serving)

- Calories: 180
- Protein: 5g
- Carbohydrates: 28g
- Fiber: 4g
- Sugars: 2g
- Fat: 7g

Servings: 4
Cooking Time: 5 minutes

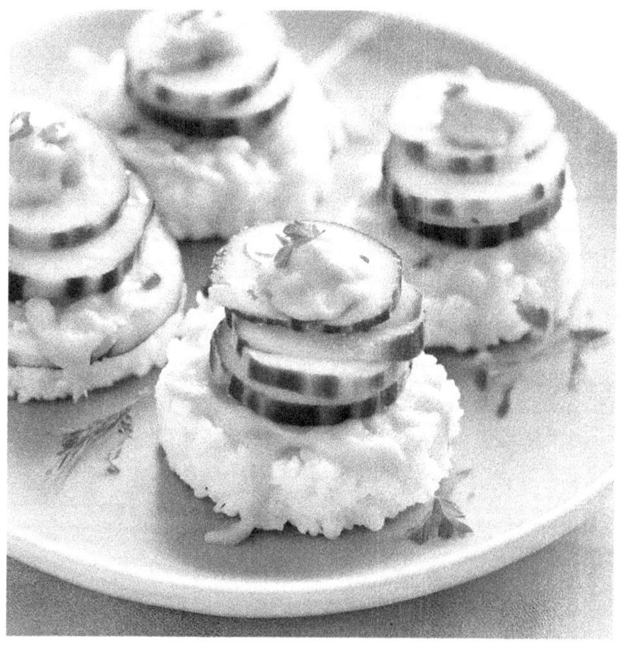

22. Coconut Yogurt with Mango and Flaxseed

Ingredients

- 2 cups coconut yogurt
- 1 ripe mango, peeled and diced
- 2 tablespoons ground flaxseed
- 1 tablespoon honey

Instructions

1. In a medium bowl, mix the coconut yogurt with the honey until well combined.
2. Divide the yogurt mixture into two bowls.
3. Top each bowl with diced mango and sprinkle with ground flaxseed.
4. Serve immediately.

Nutrition Info (Per Serving)

- Calories: 250
- Protein: 3g
- Carbohydrates: 35g
- Fiber: 6g
- Sugars: 25g
- Fat: 10g

Servings: 2
Cooking Time: 5 minutes

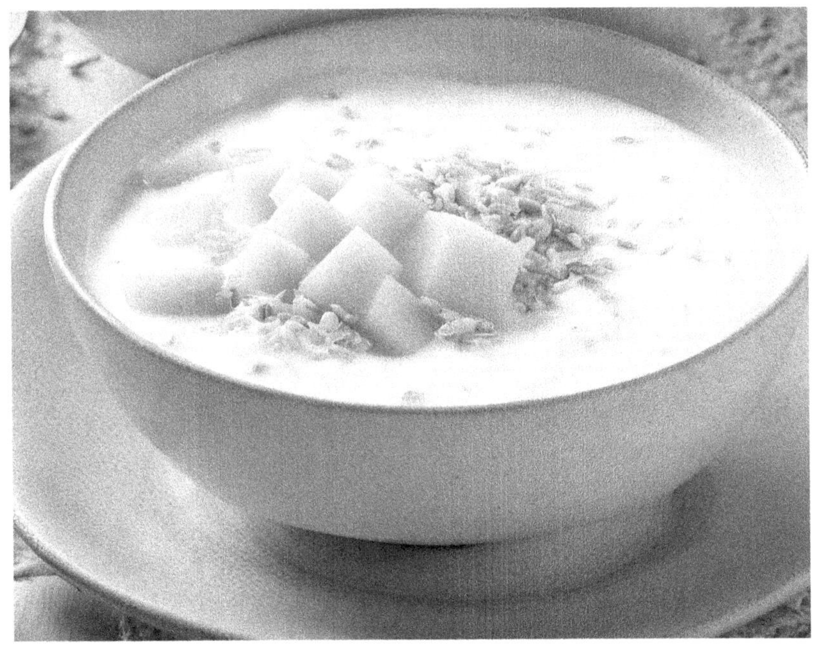

23. Oat Bran Muffins with Prunes

Ingredients

- 1 cup oat bran
- 1 cup gluten-free flour blend
- 1 teaspoon baking powder
- 1/2 teaspoon baking soda
- 1 teaspoon ground cinnamon
- 1/4 cup honey
- 1/4 cup unsweetened applesauce
- 1/4 cup olive oil
- 2 eggs
- 1 teaspoon vanilla extract
- 1 cup chopped prunes

Instructions

1. Preheat the oven to 350°F (175°C). Line a muffin tin with paper liners or grease with olive oil.
2. In a large bowl, whisk together the oat bran, gluten-free flour, baking powder, baking soda, and cinnamon.
3. In another bowl, mix the honey, applesauce, olive oil, eggs, and vanilla extract until well combined.
4. Add the wet ingredients to the dry ingredients and stir until just combined.
5. Fold in the chopped prunes.
6. Divide the batter evenly among the muffin cups.
7. Bake for 20-25 minutes, or until a toothpick inserted into the center of a muffin comes out clean.
8. Let the muffins cool slightly before serving.

Nutrition Info (Per Muffin)

- Calories: 180
- Protein: 4g
- Carbohydrates: 30g
- Fiber: 5g
- Sugars: 15g
- Fat: 6g

Servings: 12 muffins
Cooking Time: 30 minutes

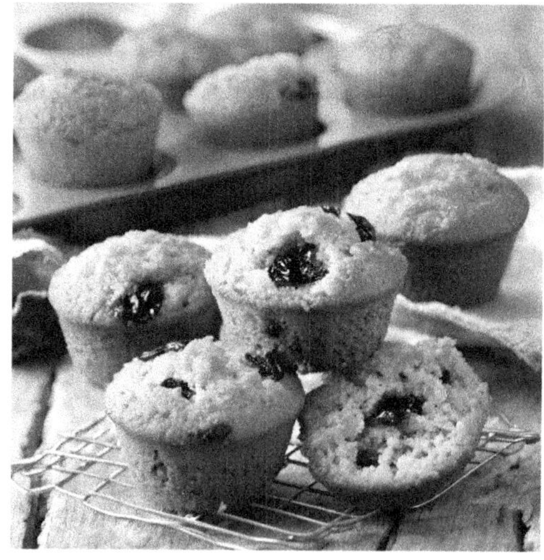

24. Gluten-Free Blueberry Waffles

Ingredients

- 1 cup gluten-free flour blend
- 1 tablespoon baking powder
- 1/2 teaspoon ground cinnamon
- 1 tablespoon honey
- 1 cup unsweetened almond milk
- 2 large eggs
- 1/4 cup melted coconut oil
- 1 cup fresh blueberries

Instructions

1. Preheat your waffle iron according to the manufacturer's instructions.
2. In a large bowl, whisk together the gluten-free flour, baking powder, and cinnamon.
3. In another bowl, mix the honey, almond milk, eggs, and melted coconut oil until well combined.
4. Add the wet ingredients to the dry ingredients and stir until just combined.
5. Fold in the blueberries.
6. Lightly grease the waffle iron with coconut oil.
7. Pour the batter onto the preheated waffle iron and cook according to the manufacturer's instructions, usually about 4-5 minutes.
8. Serve the waffles warm with additional blueberries or a drizzle of honey if desired.

Nutrition Info (Per Serving)

- Calories: 200
- Protein: 5g
- Carbohydrates: 25g
- Fiber: 3g
- Sugars: 8g
- Fat: 9g

Servings: 4

Cooking Time: 20 minutes

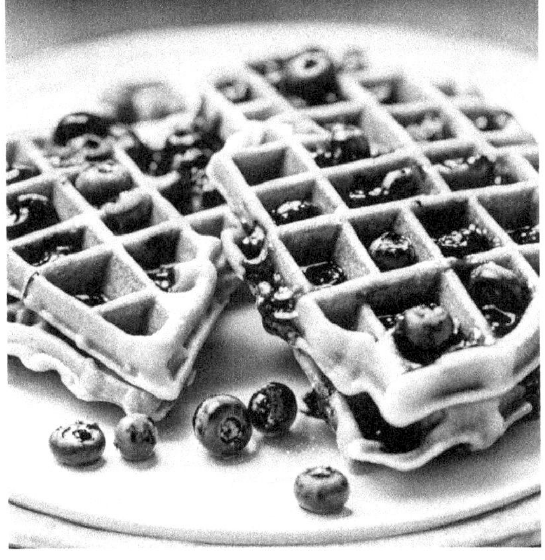

25. Kefir with Mixed Berries

Ingredients

- 2 cups plain kefir
- 1 cup mixed berries (strawberries, blueberries, raspberries)
- 1 tablespoon honey
- 1 tablespoon chia seeds

Instructions

1. In two serving glasses or bowls, divide the kefir equally.
2. Top each serving with mixed berries.
3. Drizzle with honey and sprinkle with chia seeds.
4. Serve immediately.

Nutrition Info (Per Serving)

- Calories: 180
- Protein: 7g
- Carbohydrates: 30g
- Fiber: 5g
- Sugars: 20g
- Fat: 4g

Servings: 2

Cooking Time: 5 minutes

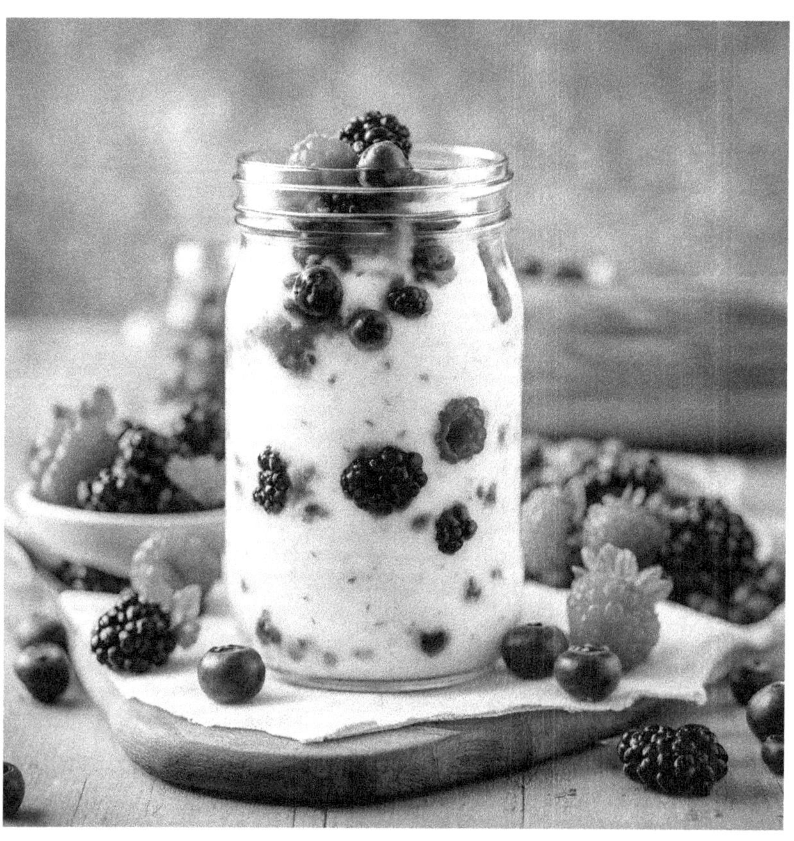

Poultry Recipes

1. Turmeric Chicken Soup

Ingredients

- 1 lb boneless, skinless chicken breasts, diced
- 1 tablespoon olive oil
- 1 large onion, chopped
- 2 garlic cloves, minced
- 1 tablespoon grated fresh ginger
- 1 tablespoon ground turmeric
- 1 teaspoon ground cumin
- 6 cups low-sodium chicken broth
- 2 carrots, sliced
- 2 celery stalks, sliced
- 1 cup kale, chopped
- 1/2 cup quinoa
- 1/4 cup fresh parsley, chopped
- Juice of 1 lemon

Instructions

1. Heat the olive oil in a large pot over medium heat. Add the onion and garlic, and cook until softened, about 5 minutes.
2. Add the ginger, turmeric, and cumin, and cook for another 2 minutes until fragrant.
3. Add the diced chicken and cook until browned on all sides.
4. Pour in the chicken broth and bring to a boil.
5. Add the carrots, celery, kale, and quinoa. Reduce the heat and simmer for 20-25 minutes, or until the vegetables and quinoa are tender.
6. Stir in the parsley and lemon juice.
7. Serve hot.

Nutrition Info (Per Serving)

- Calories: 280
- Protein: 25g
- Carbohydrates: 25g
- Fiber: 5g
- Sugars: 4g
- Fat: 10g

Servings: 4
Cooking Time: 40 minutes

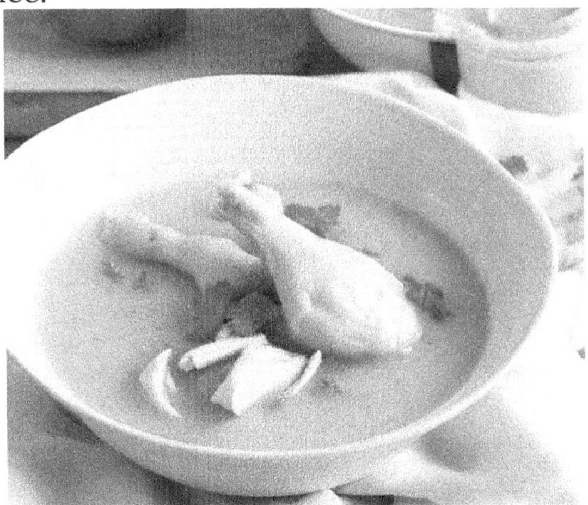

2. Grilled Chicken with Avocado Salsa

Ingredients

- 4 boneless, skinless chicken breasts
- 2 tablespoons olive oil
- 1 teaspoon ground cumin
- 1 teaspoon ground paprika
- 1 teaspoon garlic powder
- 1 avocado, diced
- 1 small tomato, diced
- 1/4 red onion, finely chopped
- 2 tablespoons fresh cilantro, chopped
- Juice of 1 lime

Instructions

1. Preheat the grill to medium-high heat.
2. In a small bowl, mix the olive oil, cumin, paprika, and garlic powder.
3. Brush the chicken breasts with the olive oil mixture.
4. Grill the chicken for 6-7 minutes on each side, or until fully cooked.
5. While the chicken is grilling, prepare the avocado salsa by combining the avocado, tomato, red onion, cilantro, and lime juice in a bowl.
6. Serve the grilled chicken topped with the avocado salsa.

Nutrition Info (Per Serving)

- Calories: 350
- Protein: 30g
- Carbohydrates: 10g
- Fiber: 5g
- Sugars: 2g
- Fat: 22g

Servings: 4
Cooking Time: 20 minutes

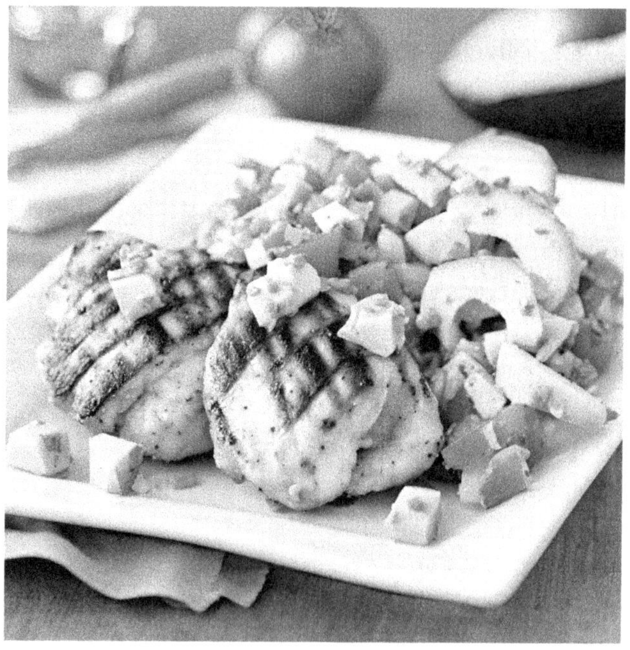

3. Slow Cooker Chicken and Sweet Potato Stew

Ingredients

- 1 lb boneless, skinless chicken thighs, cut into chunks
- 2 large sweet potatoes, peeled and diced
- 1 large onion, chopped
- 2 garlic cloves, minced
- 1 can (14.5 oz) diced tomatoes, undrained
- 2 cups low-sodium chicken broth
- 1 teaspoon ground cumin
- 1 teaspoon ground coriander
- 1/2 teaspoon ground cinnamon
- 1/4 teaspoon ground cayenne (optional)
- 1 cup baby spinach
- 1/4 cup fresh parsley, chopped

Instructions

1. Place the chicken, sweet potatoes, onion, and garlic in the slow cooker.
2. Add the diced tomatoes, chicken broth, cumin, coriander, cinnamon, and cayenne (if using).
3. Stir to combine.
4. Cover and cook on low for 6-7 hours or high for 3-4 hours, until the chicken and sweet potatoes are tender.
5. Stir in the baby spinach and let it wilt.
6. Serve the stew garnished with fresh parsley.

Nutrition Info (Per Serving)

- Calories: 300
- Protein: 25g
- Carbohydrates: 35g
- Fiber: 7g
- Sugars: 8g
- Fat: 6g

Servings: 4

Cooking Time: 7 hours (slow cooker)

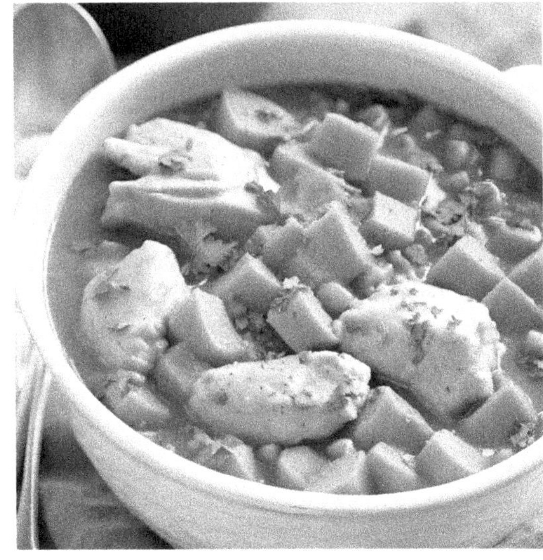

4. Chicken Salad with Walnuts and Dried Cranberries
Ingredients

- 2 cups cooked, shredded chicken breast
- 1/2 cup plain Greek yogurt
- 1 tablespoon Dijon mustard
- 1 tablespoon honey
- 1/2 cup celery, diced
- 1/2 cup walnuts, chopped
- 1/2 cup dried cranberries
- 2 green onions, sliced
- 1 tablespoon fresh parsley, chopped
- 1 teaspoon apple cider vinegar

Instructions

1. In a large bowl, combine the Greek yogurt, Dijon mustard, honey, and apple cider vinegar.
2. Add the shredded chicken, celery, walnuts, dried cranberries, green onions, and parsley.
3. Mix until well combined.
4. Serve the chicken salad on a bed of greens or as a sandwich filling.

Nutrition Info (Per Serving)

- Calories: 250
- Protein: 20g
- Carbohydrates: 15g
- Fiber: 3g
- Sugars: 10g
- Fat: 12g

Servings: 4
Cooking Time: 10 minutes

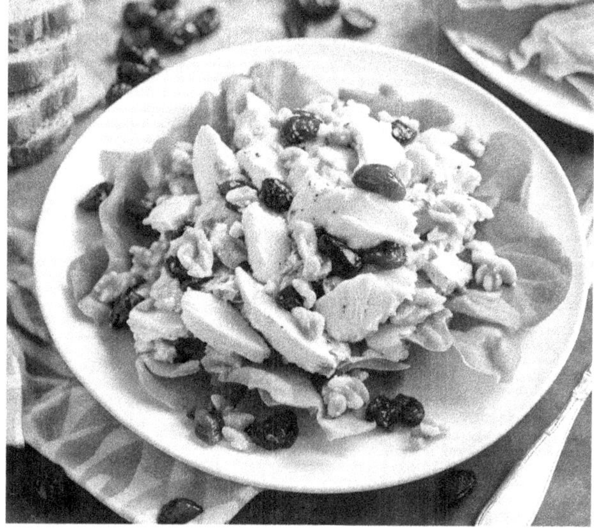

5. Ginger Chicken Stir-Fry

Ingredients

- 1 lb boneless, skinless chicken breast, thinly sliced
- 2 tablespoons olive oil
- 1 large red bell pepper, sliced
- 1 cup broccoli florets
- 1 cup snap peas
- 1 large carrot, julienned
- 2 garlic cloves, minced
- 1 tablespoon grated fresh ginger
- 1/4 cup low-sodium soy sauce or tamari
- 1 tablespoon honey
- 1 tablespoon rice vinegar
- 1 teaspoon sesame oil
- 2 green onions, sliced
- 1 tablespoon sesame seeds (optional)

Instructions

1. Heat the olive oil in a large skillet or wok over medium-high heat.
2. Add the sliced chicken and cook until browned and cooked through, about 5-7 minutes.
3. Remove the chicken from the skillet and set aside.
4. In the same skillet, add the bell pepper, broccoli, snap peas, and carrot. Stir-fry for 3-4 minutes until tender-crisp.
5. Add the garlic and ginger, and stir-fry for another minute.
6. Return the chicken to the skillet.
7. In a small bowl, mix the soy sauce, honey, rice vinegar, and sesame oil. Pour over the chicken and vegetables.
8. Stir well to combine and cook for another 2-3 minutes until everything is heated through.
9. Garnish with sliced green onions and sesame seeds, if using.
10. Serve hot.

Nutrition Info (Per Serving)

- Calories: 300
- Protein: 30g
- Carbohydrates: 18g
- Fiber: 4g
- Sugars: 10g
- Fat: 12g

Servings: 4

Cooking Time: 20 minutes

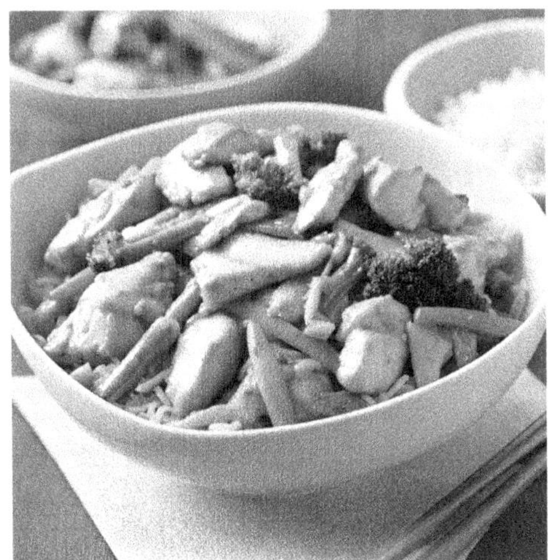

6. Chicken and Spinach Stuffed Sweet Peppers

Ingredients

- 4 large sweet bell peppers, halved and seeded
- 1 lb ground chicken
- 1 tablespoon olive oil
- 1 small onion, finely chopped
- 2 garlic cloves, minced
- 1 cup fresh spinach, chopped
- 1/2 cup cooked quinoa
- 1 teaspoon dried oregano
- 1/2 teaspoon ground cumin
- 1/2 cup grated Parmesan cheese

Instructions

1. Preheat the oven to 375°F (190°C).
2. In a large skillet, heat the olive oil over medium heat. Add the onion and garlic, and cook until softened, about 5 minutes.
3. Add the ground chicken and cook until browned, breaking it up with a spoon as it cooks.
4. Stir in the spinach, cooked quinoa, oregano, and cumin. Cook for another 2-3 minutes until the spinach is wilted.
5. Remove from heat and stir in the grated Parmesan cheese.
6. Place the halved bell peppers in a baking dish and stuff them with the chicken and spinach mixture.
7. Cover the dish with foil and bake for 30 minutes.
8. Remove the foil and bake for an additional 10 minutes, until the peppers are tender and the filling is golden.
9. Serve warm.

Nutrition Info (Per Serving)

- Calories: 280
- Protein: 25g
- Carbohydrates: 20g
- Fiber: 4g
- Sugars: 6g
- Fat: 12g

Servings: 4
Cooking Time: 45 minutes

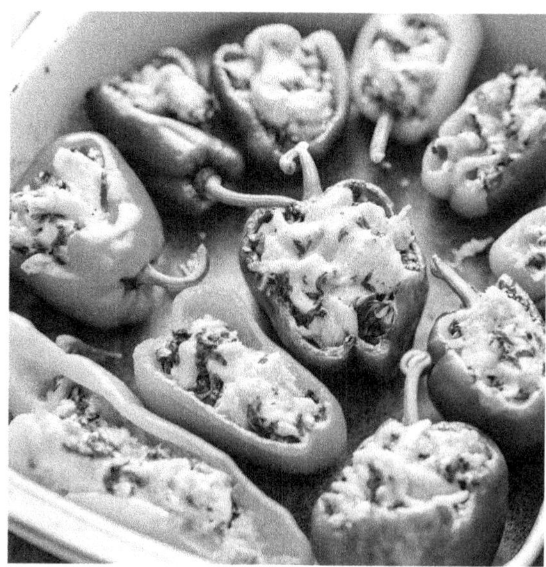

7. Baked Lemon and Herb Chicken

Ingredients

- 4 boneless, skinless chicken breasts
- 2 tablespoons olive oil
- Juice of 2 lemons
- Zest of 1 lemon
- 2 garlic cloves, minced
- 1 tablespoon fresh thyme, chopped
- 1 tablespoon fresh rosemary, chopped
- 1/4 teaspoon ground paprika

Instructions

1. Preheat the oven to 375°F (190°C).
2. In a small bowl, mix together the olive oil, lemon juice, lemon zest, garlic, thyme, rosemary, and paprika.
3. Place the chicken breasts in a baking dish and pour the lemon and herb mixture over them, ensuring they are well coated.
4. Cover the dish with foil and bake for 25 minutes.
5. Remove the foil and bake for an additional 10 minutes, until the chicken is cooked through and the top is lightly browned.
6. Serve warm.

Nutrition Info (Per Serving)

- Calories: 250
- Protein: 30g
- Carbohydrates: 3g
- Fiber: 1g
- Sugars: 1g
- Fat: 12g

Servings: 4
Cooking Time: 35 minutes

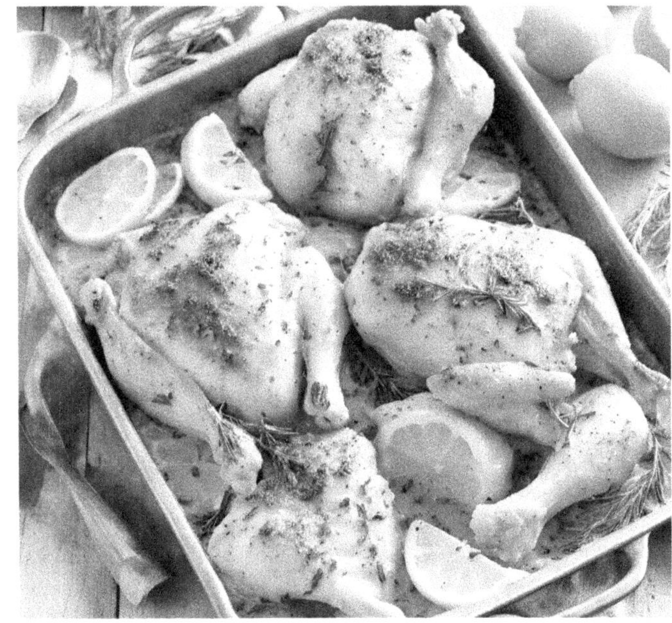

8. Chicken and Barley Soup

Ingredients

- 1 lb boneless, skinless chicken thighs, cut into chunks
- 1 tablespoon olive oil
- 1 large onion, chopped
- 2 garlic cloves, minced
- 3 carrots, sliced
- 3 celery stalks, sliced
- 1 cup pearl barley
- 8 cups low-sodium chicken broth
- 1 teaspoon dried thyme
- 1 teaspoon dried oregano
- 2 cups fresh spinach, chopped

Instructions

1. In a large pot, heat the olive oil over medium heat. Add the onion and garlic, and cook until softened, about 5 minutes.
2. Add the chicken chunks and cook until browned on all sides.
3. Stir in the carrots, celery, and barley.
4. Pour in the chicken broth and add the thyme and oregano. Bring to a boil.
5. Reduce the heat and simmer for 45 minutes, or until the barley is tender.
6. Stir in the chopped spinach and cook for an additional 5 minutes until wilted.
7. Serve hot.

Nutrition Info (Per Serving)

- Calories: 300
- Protein: 25g
- Carbohydrates: 40g
- Fiber: 8g
- Sugars: 5g
- Fat: 7g

Servings: 6

Cooking Time: 1 hour

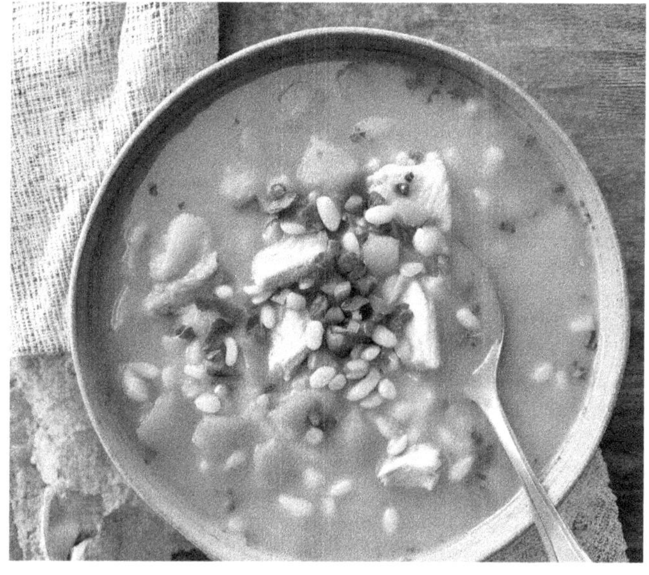

9. Cilantro Lime Chicken Skewers

Ingredients

- 1 lb boneless, skinless chicken breasts, cut into 1-inch pieces
- 1/4 cup olive oil
- Juice of 2 limes
- Zest of 1 lime
- 2 garlic cloves, minced
- 1/4 cup fresh cilantro, chopped
- 1 teaspoon ground cumin

Instructions

1. In a large bowl, whisk together the olive oil, lime juice, lime zest, garlic, cilantro, and cumin.
2. Add the chicken pieces and toss to coat. Marinate in the refrigerator for at least 30 minutes, up to 2 hours.
3. Preheat the grill to medium-high heat.
4. Thread the marinated chicken pieces onto skewers.
5. Grill the chicken skewers for 6-8 minutes on each side, or until the chicken is fully cooked.
6. Serve warm.

Nutrition Info (Per Serving)

- Calories: 220
- Protein: 25g
- Carbohydrates: 2g
- Fiber: 0g
- Sugars: 0g
- Fat: 12g

Servings: 4

Cooking Time: 20 minutes (plus marinating time)

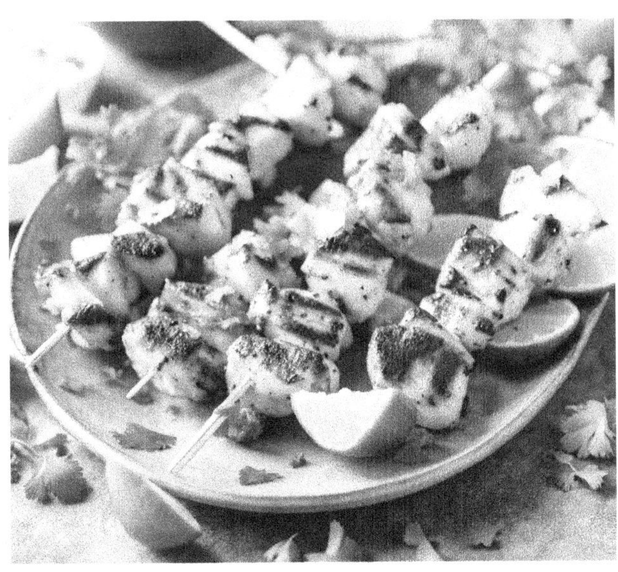

10. Chicken Quinoa Salad with Olive Oil Dressing

Ingredients

- 1 lb boneless, skinless chicken breasts, grilled and sliced
- 1 cup quinoa
- 2 cups water
- 1 cup cherry tomatoes, halved
- 1 cucumber, diced
- 1/4 red onion, finely chopped
- 1/4 cup fresh parsley, chopped
- 1/4 cup olive oil
- Juice of 1 lemon
- 1 garlic clove, minced

Instructions

1. Rinse the quinoa under cold water.
2. In a medium saucepan, bring the water to a boil. Add the quinoa, reduce heat to low, cover, and simmer for 15 minutes or until the water is absorbed and the quinoa is tender.
3. In a large bowl, combine the cooked quinoa, cherry tomatoes, cucumber, red onion, and parsley.
4. In a small bowl, whisk together the olive oil, lemon juice, and minced garlic.
5. Pour the dressing over the quinoa salad and toss to combine.
6. Top with the grilled chicken slices.
7. Serve warm or chilled.

Nutrition Info (Per Serving)

- Calories: 350
- Protein: 28g
- Carbohydrates: 28g
- Fiber: 5g
- Sugars: 4g
- Fat: 15g

Servings: 4
Cooking Time: 30 minutes

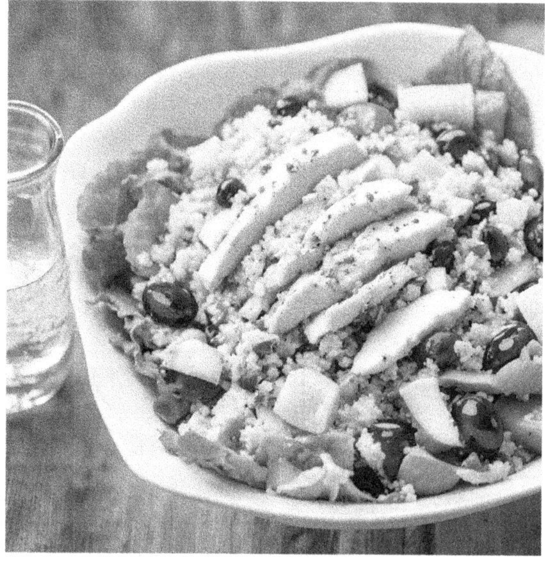

11. Greek Yogurt Chicken Alfredo with Gluten-Free Pasta

Ingredients

- 1 lb boneless, skinless chicken breasts, cut into bite-sized pieces
- 2 tablespoons olive oil
- 12 oz gluten-free pasta
- 1 cup Greek yogurt
- 1/2 cup grated Parmesan cheese
- 2 garlic cloves, minced
- 1 cup low-sodium chicken broth
- 1 tablespoon lemon juice
- 1/4 teaspoon ground nutmeg
- 2 tablespoons fresh parsley, chopped

Instructions

1. Cook the gluten-free pasta according to package instructions. Drain and set aside.
2. In a large skillet, heat the olive oil over medium heat. Add the chicken pieces and cook until browned and cooked through, about 7-10 minutes. Remove from skillet and set aside.
3. In the same skillet, add the garlic and cook for 1-2 minutes until fragrant.
4. Stir in the chicken broth and bring to a simmer.
5. Reduce heat and stir in the Greek yogurt, Parmesan cheese, lemon juice, and ground nutmeg. Mix until smooth and creamy.
6. Add the cooked chicken and pasta to the skillet and toss to combine.
7. Garnish with fresh parsley and serve warm.

Nutrition Info (Per Serving)

- Calories: 400
- Protein: 30g
- Carbohydrates: 45g
- Fiber: 3g
- Sugars: 4g
- Fat: 12g

Servings: 4
Cooking Time: 30 minutes

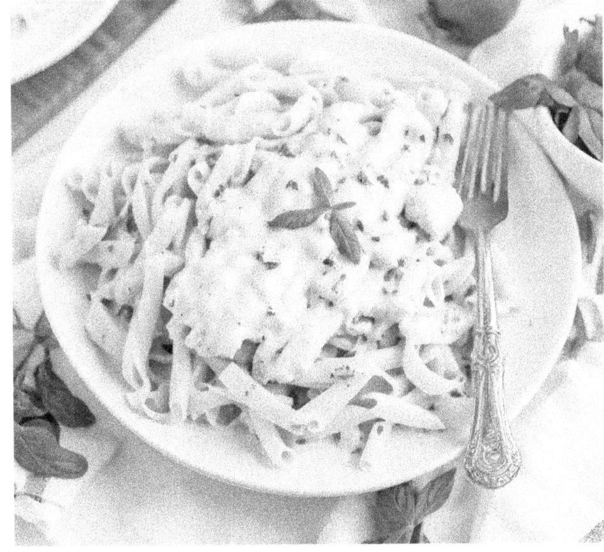

12. Roasted Chicken with Root Vegetables

Ingredients

- 1 whole chicken (about 4 lbs)
- 2 tablespoons olive oil
- 2 large carrots, peeled and chopped
- 2 parsnips, peeled and chopped
- 1 large sweet potato, peeled and chopped
- 1 large onion, quartered
- 4 garlic cloves, minced
- 1 tablespoon fresh thyme, chopped
- 1 tablespoon fresh rosemary, chopped
- Juice of 1 lemon

Instructions

1. Preheat the oven to 375°F (190°C).
2. Rub the chicken with olive oil, garlic, thyme, rosemary, and lemon juice.
3. Place the chicken in a large roasting pan.
4. Arrange the carrots, parsnips, sweet potato, and onion around the chicken.
5. Roast for 1 hour and 30 minutes, or until the chicken reaches an internal temperature of 165°F (75°C) and the vegetables are tender.
6. Let the chicken rest for 10 minutes before carving.
7. Serve warm with roasted vegetables.

Nutrition Info (Per Serving)

- Calories: 450
- Protein: 40g
- Carbohydrates: 30g
- Fiber: 6g
- Sugars: 10g
- Fat: 18g

Servings: 6

Cooking Time: 1 hour 40 minutes

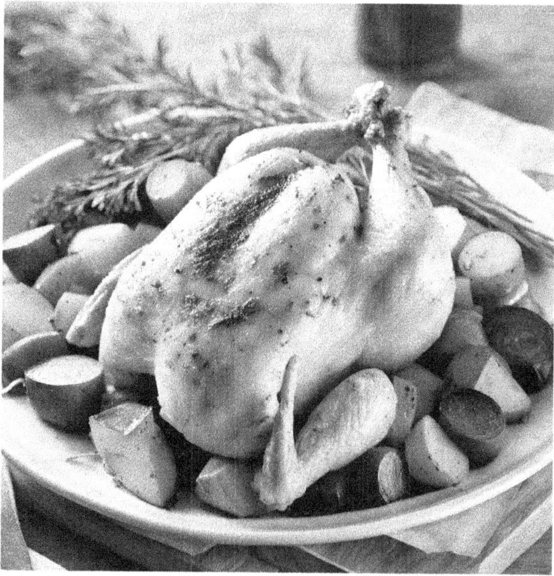

13. Basil and Pine Nut Chicken Patties

Ingredients

- 1 lb ground chicken
- 1/4 cup fresh basil, chopped
- 1/4 cup pine nuts, toasted and chopped
- 1/4 cup grated Parmesan cheese
- 1 garlic clove, minced
- 1 egg
- 2 tablespoons olive oil

Instructions

1. In a large bowl, combine the ground chicken, basil, pine nuts, Parmesan cheese, garlic, and egg. Mix until well combined.
2. Form the mixture into 4 patties.
3. Heat the olive oil in a large skillet over medium heat.
4. Cook the patties for 5-6 minutes on each side, or until browned and cooked through.
5. Serve warm.

Nutrition Info (Per Serving)

- Calories: 250
- Protein: 25g
- Carbohydrates: 3g
- Fiber: 1g
- Sugars: 0g
- Fat: 16g

Servings: 4
Cooking Time: 20 minutes

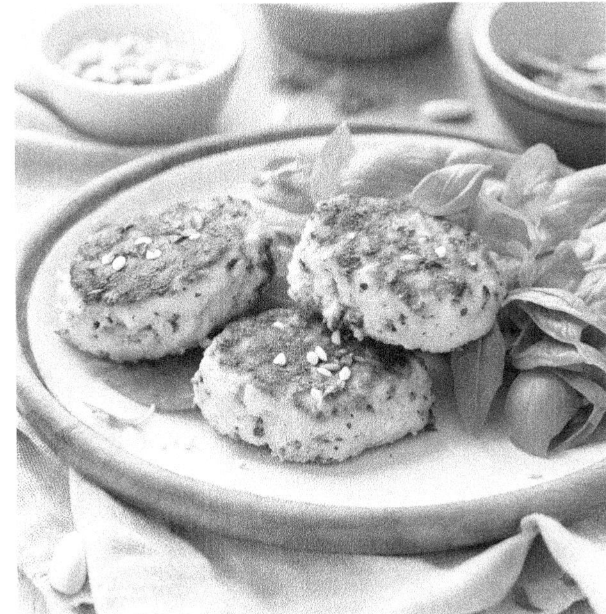

14. Chicken and Vegetable Kabobs

Ingredients

- 1 lb boneless, skinless chicken breasts, cut into 1-inch pieces
- 2 bell peppers (any color), cut into 1-inch pieces
- 1 large red onion, cut into wedges
- 1 zucchini, sliced
- 1/4 cup olive oil
- Juice of 2 lemons
- 1 tablespoon dried oregano
- 1 tablespoon garlic powder

Instructions

1. Preheat the grill to medium-high heat.
2. In a large bowl, whisk together the olive oil, lemon juice, oregano, and garlic powder.
3. Add the chicken pieces and vegetables to the bowl, tossing to coat.
4. Thread the chicken and vegetables onto skewers, alternating between them.
5. Grill the kabobs for 10-12 minutes, turning occasionally, until the chicken is fully cooked and the vegetables are tender.
6. Serve warm.

Nutrition Info (Per Serving)

- Calories: 300
- Protein: 25g
- Carbohydrates: 10g
- Fiber: 3g
- Sugars: 4g
- Fat: 18g

Servings: 4
Cooking Time: 20 minutes

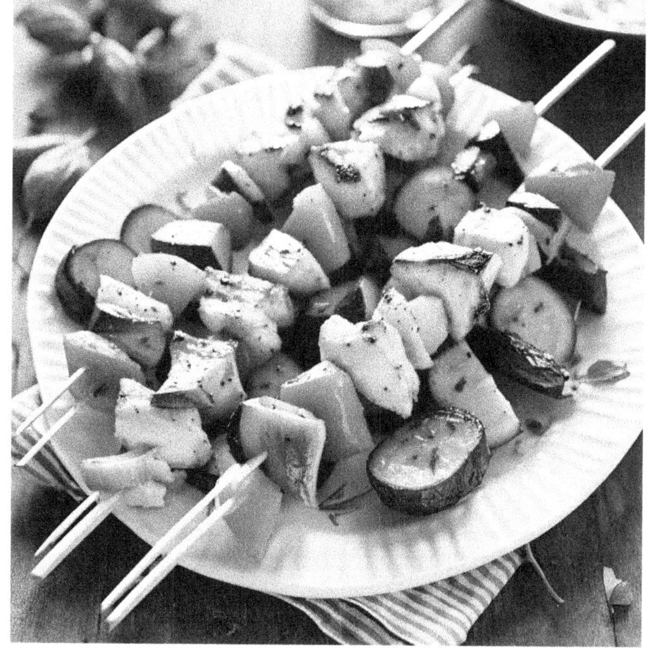

15. Chicken Piccata with Capers

Ingredients

- 4 boneless, skinless chicken breasts
- 1/4 cup almond flour
- 2 tablespoons olive oil
- 1/4 cup lemon juice
- 1/2 cup low-sodium chicken broth
- 1/4 cup capers, rinsed and drained
- 2 tablespoons fresh parsley, chopped

Instructions

1. Place the chicken breasts between two sheets of plastic wrap and pound to 1/2-inch thickness.
2. Dredge the chicken in almond flour, shaking off any excess.
3. Heat the olive oil in a large skillet over medium-high heat.
4. Add the chicken breasts and cook for 4-5 minutes on each side, until golden brown and cooked through. Remove the chicken from the skillet and set aside.
5. In the same skillet, add the lemon juice, chicken broth, and capers. Bring to a boil and cook for 2 minutes, until the sauce is slightly reduced.
6. Return the chicken to the skillet and spoon the sauce over the top.
7. Garnish with fresh parsley and serve warm.

Nutrition Info (Per Serving)

- Calories: 320
- Protein: 30g
- Carbohydrates: 6g
- Fiber: 2g
- Sugars: 1g
- Fat: 20g

Servings: 4
Cooking Time: 20 minutes

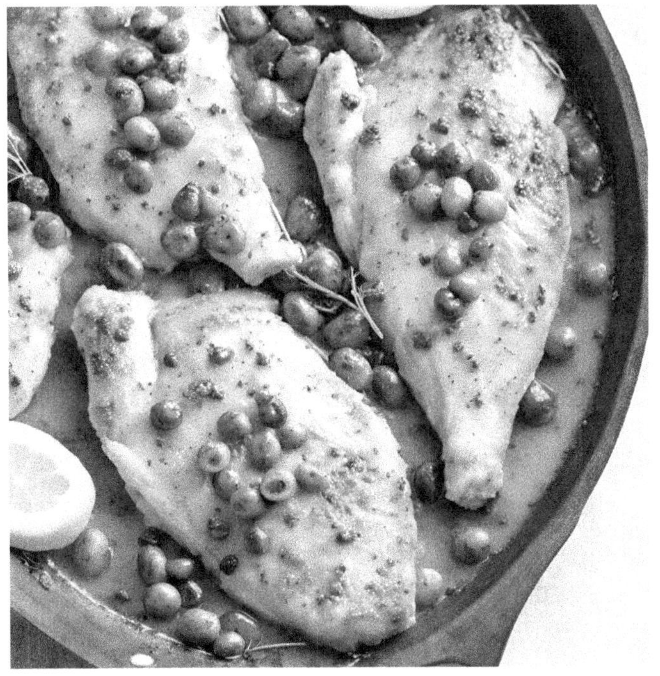

16. Creamy Chicken and Mushroom Soup

Ingredients

- 1 lb boneless, skinless chicken thighs, cut into chunks
- 2 tablespoons olive oil
- 1 large onion, chopped
- 3 garlic cloves, minced
- 2 cups sliced mushrooms
- 4 cups low-sodium chicken broth
- 1 cup unsweetened almond milk
- 1 teaspoon dried thyme
- 1 teaspoon dried rosemary
- 2 tablespoons cornstarch mixed with 2 tablespoons water (slurry)
- 1/4 cup fresh parsley, chopped

Instructions

1. In a large pot, heat the olive oil over medium heat. Add the onion and garlic, and cook until softened, about 5 minutes.
2. Add the chicken and cook until browned.
3. Add the mushrooms and cook for another 5 minutes.
4. Pour in the chicken broth and bring to a boil.
5. Reduce the heat and simmer for 20 minutes.
6. Stir in the almond milk, thyme, rosemary, and cornstarch slurry. Cook until the soup thickens, about 5 minutes.
7. Garnish with fresh parsley and serve warm.

Nutrition Info (Per Serving)

- Calories: 250
- Protein: 22g
- Carbohydrates: 10g
- Fiber: 2g
- Sugars: 2g
- Fat: 14g

Servings: 4
Cooking Time: 40 minutes

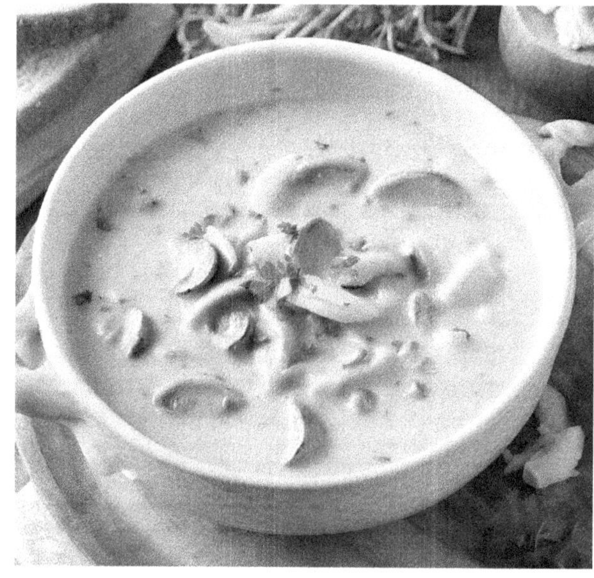

17. Chicken and Apple Sausages

Ingredients

- 1 lb ground chicken
- 1 apple, peeled and grated
- 1/2 onion, finely chopped
- 2 garlic cloves, minced
- 1 tablespoon fresh sage, chopped
- 1 teaspoon dried thyme
- 1/4 teaspoon ground allspice
- 1 tablespoon olive oil

Instructions

1. In a large bowl, combine the ground chicken, grated apple, onion, garlic, sage, thyme, and allspice. Mix until well combined.
2. Form the mixture into small patties or sausages.
3. Heat the olive oil in a large skillet over medium heat.
4. Cook the sausages for 4-5 minutes on each side, or until browned and cooked through.
5. Serve warm.

Nutrition Info (Per Serving)

- Calories: 210
- Protein: 25g
- Carbohydrates: 6g
- Fiber: 1g
- Sugars: 4g
- Fat: 10g

Servings: 4
Cooking Time: 20 minutes

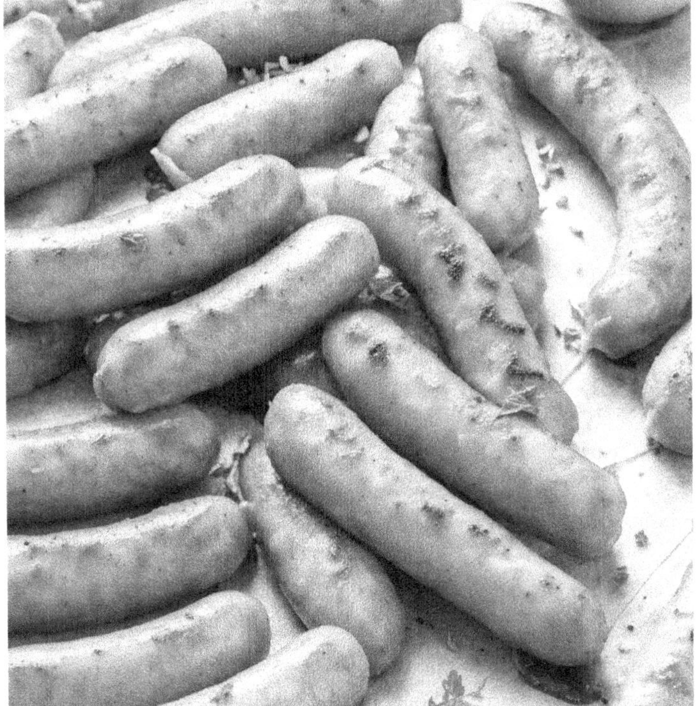

18. Pesto Chicken Flatbread with Gluten-Free Base

Ingredients

- 2 gluten-free flatbreads
- 1 lb boneless, skinless chicken breasts, cooked and sliced
- 1/2 cup basil pesto (store-bought or homemade)
- 1/2 cup cherry tomatoes, halved
- 1/4 cup red onion, thinly sliced
- 1/4 cup grated Parmesan cheese
- 1/4 cup fresh basil leaves, chopped

Instructions

1. Preheat the oven to 400°F (200°C).
2. Place the gluten-free flatbreads on a baking sheet.
3. Spread 1/4 cup of pesto on each flatbread.
4. Top with sliced chicken, cherry tomatoes, red onion, and Parmesan cheese.
5. Bake for 10-12 minutes, or until the flatbreads are crispy and the cheese is melted.
6. Garnish with fresh basil leaves.
7. Serve warm.

Nutrition Info (Per Serving)

- Calories: 350
- Protein: 30g
- Carbohydrates: 25g
- Fiber: 3g
- Sugars: 2g
- Fat: 15g

Servings: 4
Cooking Time: 20 minutes

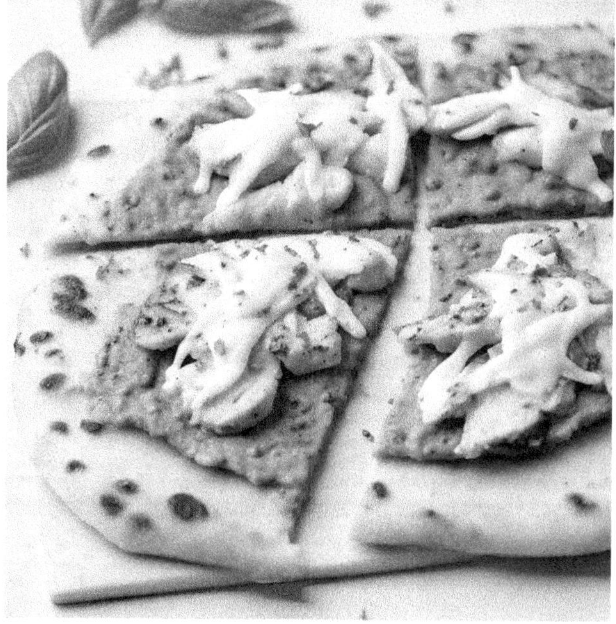

19. Chicken Paillard with Arugula Salad

Ingredients

- 4 boneless, skinless chicken breasts, pounded thin
- 2 tablespoons olive oil
- Juice of 1 lemon
- 1 garlic clove, minced
- 4 cups arugula
- 1/2 cup cherry tomatoes, halved
- 1/4 cup red onion, thinly sliced
- 1/4 cup shaved Parmesan cheese

Instructions

1. In a large skillet, heat the olive oil over medium-high heat.
2. Add the chicken breasts and cook for 3-4 minutes on each side, until golden brown and cooked through. Remove from skillet and set aside.
3. In a small bowl, whisk together the lemon juice and minced garlic.
4. In a large bowl, toss the arugula, cherry tomatoes, red onion, and Parmesan cheese with the lemon juice mixture.
5. Serve the chicken paillard topped with the arugula salad.

Nutrition Info (Per Serving)

- Calories: 300
- Protein: 35g
- Carbohydrates: 6g
- Fiber: 2g
- Sugars: 2g
- Fat: 15g

Servings: 4

Cooking Time: 15 minutes

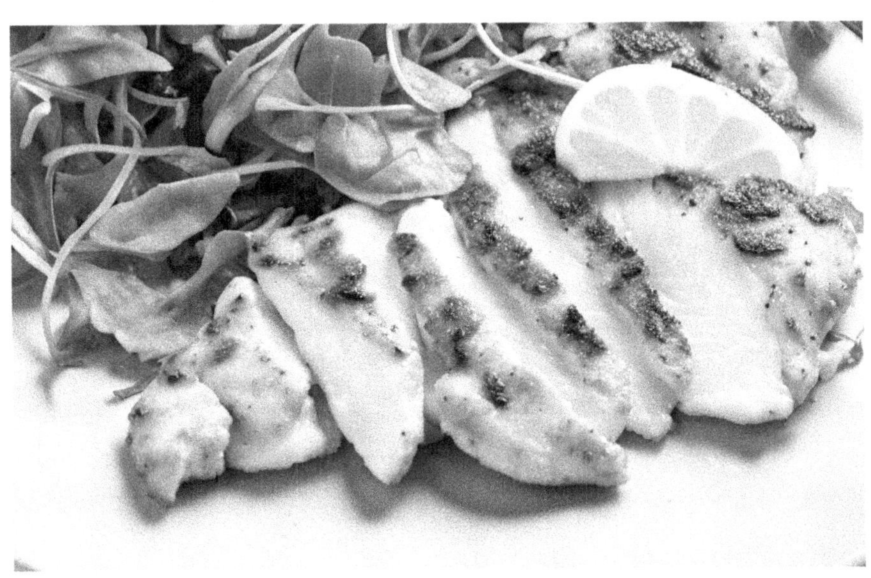

20. Chicken Gumbo with Okra

Ingredients

- 1 lb boneless, skinless chicken thighs, cut into chunks
- 2 tablespoons olive oil
- 1 large onion, chopped
- 1 green bell pepper, chopped
- 2 celery stalks, chopped
- 3 garlic cloves, minced
- 1 can (14.5 oz) diced tomatoes, undrained
- 4 cups low-sodium chicken broth
- 2 cups sliced okra (fresh or frozen)
- 1 teaspoon dried thyme
- 1/2 teaspoon ground paprika
- 1/4 teaspoon cayenne pepper (optional)
- 2 cups cooked brown rice

Instructions

1. In a large pot, heat the olive oil over medium heat. Add the onion, bell pepper, and celery, and cook until softened, about 5 minutes.
2. Add the garlic and cook for another minute.
3. Stir in the chicken chunks and cook until browned.
4. Add the diced tomatoes, chicken broth, okra, thyme, paprika, and cayenne pepper (if using). Bring to a boil.
5. Reduce the heat and simmer for 30 minutes, or until the chicken is cooked through and the vegetables are tender.
6. Serve the gumbo over cooked brown rice.

Nutrition Info (Per Serving)

- Calories: 350
- Protein: 25g
- Carbohydrates: 35g
- Fiber: 5g
- Sugars: 5g
- Fat: 12g

Servings: 4

Cooking Time: 45 minutes

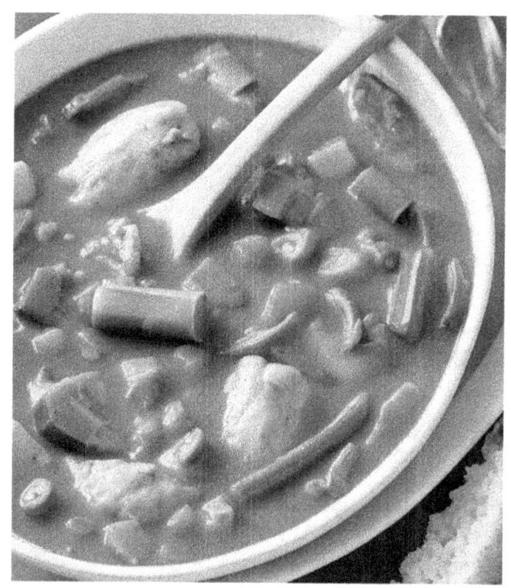

21. Chicken Stir-Fry with Broccoli and Almonds

Ingredients

- 1 lb boneless, skinless chicken breasts, thinly sliced
- 2 tablespoons olive oil
- 2 cups broccoli florets
- 1 red bell pepper, sliced
- 1 carrot, julienned
- 1/4 cup sliced almonds
- 2 garlic cloves, minced
- 1 tablespoon grated fresh ginger
- 1/4 cup low-sodium soy sauce or tamari
- 1 tablespoon honey
- 1 tablespoon rice vinegar

Instructions

1. Heat 1 tablespoon of olive oil in a large skillet or wok over medium-high heat.
2. Add the sliced chicken and cook until browned and cooked through, about 5-7 minutes. Remove the chicken from the skillet and set aside.
3. Add the remaining tablespoon of olive oil to the skillet.
4. Add the broccoli, red bell pepper, and carrot, and stir-fry for 4-5 minutes until the vegetables are tender-crisp.
5. Add the garlic and ginger, and stir-fry for another minute.
6. In a small bowl, mix the soy sauce, honey, and rice vinegar.
7. Return the chicken to the skillet and pour the sauce over the chicken and vegetables. Stir to combine and cook for another 2-3 minutes until heated through.
8. Sprinkle with sliced almonds before serving.

Nutrition Info (Per Serving)

- Calories: 300
- Protein: 25g
- Carbohydrates: 18g
- Fiber: 4g
- Sugars: 8g
- Fat: 14g

Servings: 4
Cooking Time: 20 minutes

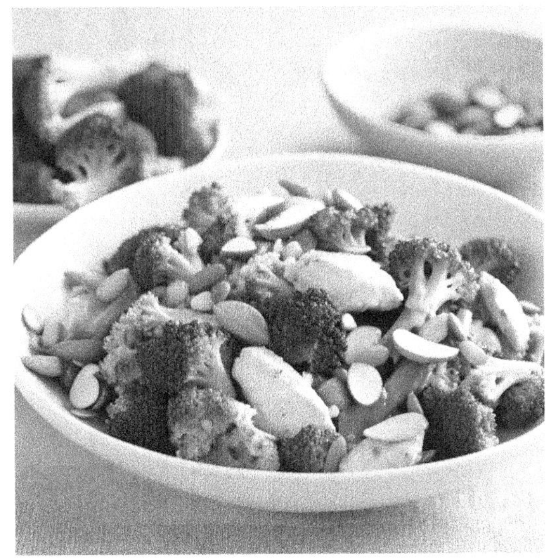

22. Poached Chicken Breast with Ginger Soy Sauce

Ingredients

- 4 boneless, skinless chicken breasts
- 4 cups low-sodium chicken broth
- 2 garlic cloves, minced
- 1 tablespoon grated fresh ginger
- 1/4 cup low-sodium soy sauce or tamari
- 1 tablespoon rice vinegar
- 1 tablespoon honey
- 2 green onions, thinly sliced

Instructions

1. In a large pot, bring the chicken broth to a boil. Add the chicken breasts, reduce the heat to low, and simmer for 15-20 minutes, or until the chicken is cooked through.
2. Remove the chicken breasts from the broth and let them cool slightly before slicing.
3. In a small bowl, mix the garlic, ginger, soy sauce, rice vinegar, and honey.
4. Drizzle the ginger soy sauce over the sliced chicken breasts.
5. Garnish with green onions.
6. Serve warm.

Nutrition Info (Per Serving)

- Calories: 200
- Protein: 30g
- Carbohydrates: 6g
- Fiber: 0g
- Sugars: 5g
- Fat: 4g

Servings: 4
Cooking Time: 25 minutes

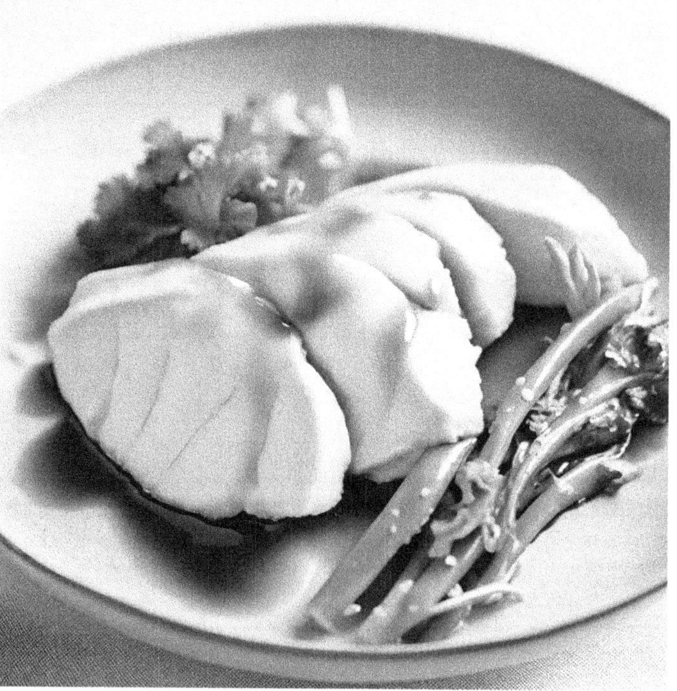

23. Honey Mustard Chicken Thighs

Ingredients

- 8 boneless, skinless chicken thighs
- 2 tablespoons olive oil
- 1/4 cup Dijon mustard
- 1/4 cup honey
- 2 garlic cloves, minced
- 1 tablespoon fresh thyme, chopped

Instructions

1. Preheat the oven to 375°F (190°C).
2. In a small bowl, mix the Dijon mustard, honey, garlic, and fresh thyme.
3. In a large oven-safe skillet, heat the olive oil over medium heat. Add the chicken thighs and cook for 4-5 minutes on each side, until browned.
4. Pour the honey mustard mixture over the chicken thighs.
5. Transfer the skillet to the oven and bake for 20-25 minutes, or until the chicken is cooked through.
6. Serve warm.

Nutrition Info (Per Serving)

- Calories: 320
- Protein: 28g
- Carbohydrates: 10g
- Fiber: 1g
- Sugars: 8g
- Fat: 18g

Servings: 4
Cooking Time: 35 minutes

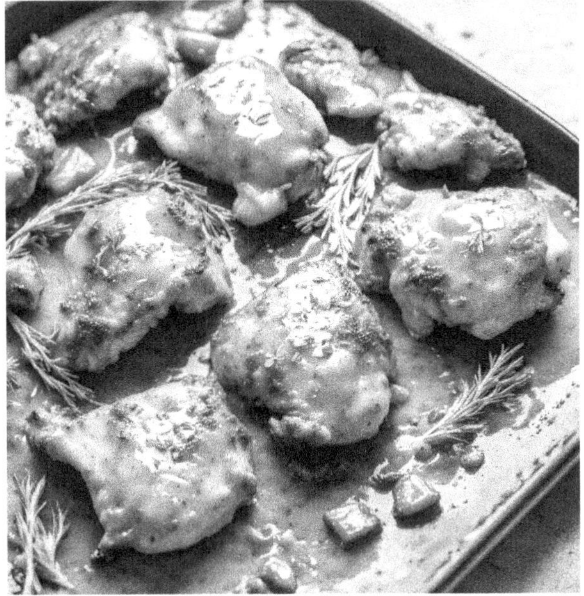

24. Sesame Ginger Turkey Wraps

Ingredients

- 1 lb ground turkey
- 2 tablespoons olive oil
- 1 garlic clove, minced
- 1 tablespoon grated fresh ginger
- 2 tablespoons low-sodium soy sauce or tamari
- 1 tablespoon rice vinegar
- 1 tablespoon honey
- 1 tablespoon sesame oil
- 4 large lettuce leaves (for wraps)
- 1/2 cup shredded carrots
- 1/2 cup cucumber, julienned
- 1/4 cup chopped fresh cilantro
- 1 tablespoon sesame seeds

Instructions

1. In a large skillet, heat the olive oil over medium heat. Add the ground turkey and cook until browned and cooked through, about 7-10 minutes.
2. Add the garlic and ginger, and cook for another minute.
3. In a small bowl, mix the soy sauce, rice vinegar, honey, and sesame oil. Pour the sauce over the turkey mixture and stir to combine. Cook for an additional 2-3 minutes until heated through.
4. Spoon the turkey mixture onto large lettuce leaves.
5. Top with shredded carrots, cucumber, cilantro, and sesame seeds.
6. Serve immediately.

Nutrition Info (Per Serving)

- Calories: 250
- Protein: 24g
- Carbohydrates: 10g
- Fiber: 2g
- Sugars: 5g
- Fat: 14g

Servings: 4

Cooking Time: 20 minutes

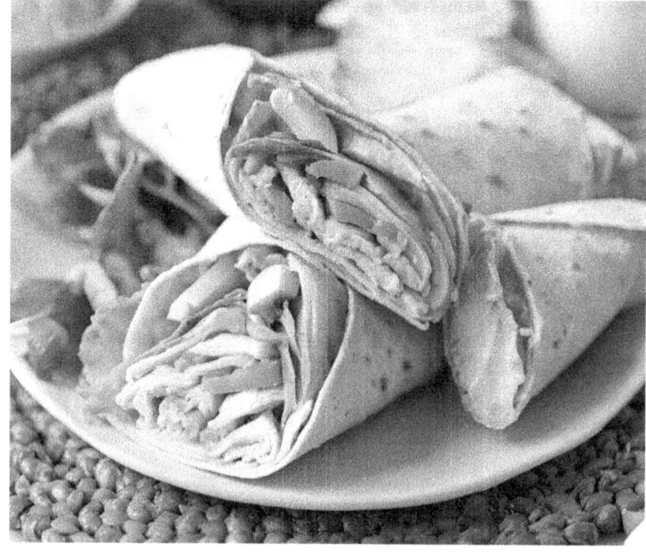

Fish and Seafood Recipes

1. Grilled Salmon with Dill and Lemon

Ingredients

- 4 salmon fillets (about 6 oz each)
- 2 tablespoons olive oil
- 2 tablespoons fresh dill, chopped
- 1 lemon, sliced
- 2 garlic cloves, minced
- Juice of 1 lemon

Instructions

1. Preheat the grill to medium-high heat.
2. In a small bowl, mix the olive oil, dill, minced garlic, and lemon juice.
3. Brush the salmon fillets with the olive oil mixture.
4. Place the salmon fillets on the grill, skin-side down. Grill for 4-5 minutes on each side, or until the salmon is cooked through and flakes easily with a fork.
5. Remove the salmon from the grill and garnish with lemon slices.
6. Serve warm.

Nutrition Info (Per Serving)

- Calories: 350
- Protein: 34g
- Carbohydrates: 2g
- Fiber: 1g
- Sugars: 0g
- Fat: 22g

Servings: 4
Cooking Time: 15 minutes

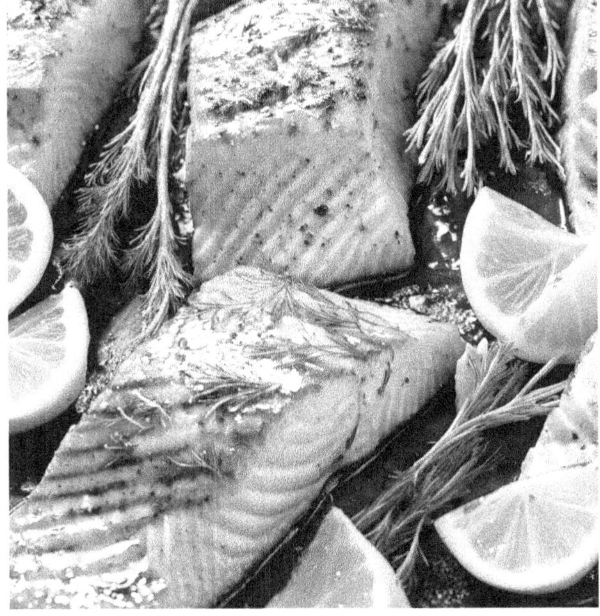

2. Shrimp and Avocado Salad

Ingredients

- 1 lb cooked shrimp, peeled and deveined
- 2 avocados, diced
- 1 cup cherry tomatoes, halved
- 1/4 red onion, finely chopped
- 1/4 cup fresh cilantro, chopped
- 2 tablespoons olive oil
- Juice of 2 limes
- 1 garlic clove, minced

Instructions

1. In a large bowl, combine the shrimp, avocados, cherry tomatoes, red onion, and cilantro.
2. In a small bowl, whisk together the olive oil, lime juice, and minced garlic.
3. Pour the dressing over the shrimp mixture and toss gently to combine.
4. Serve immediately or refrigerate until ready to serve.

Nutrition Info (Per Serving)

- Calories: 300
- Protein: 25g
- Carbohydrates: 12g
- Fiber: 7g
- Sugars: 3g
- Fat: 18g

Servings: 4
Cooking Time: 10 minutes

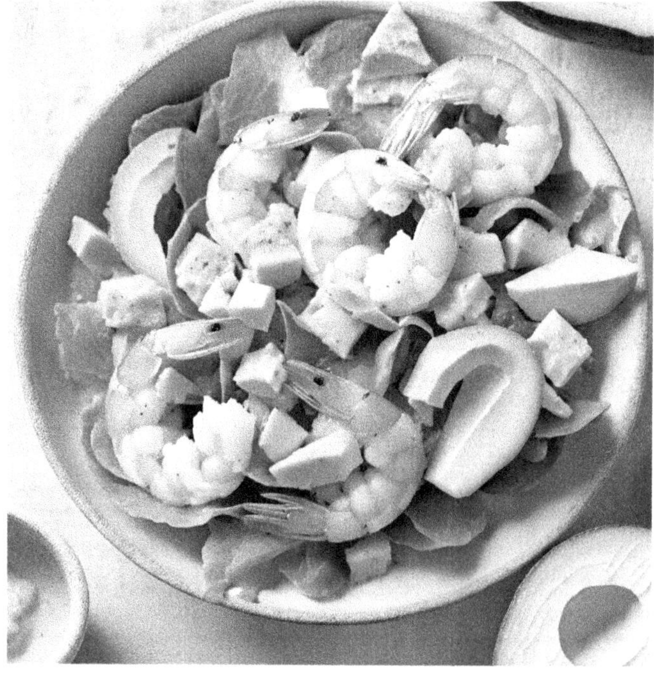

3. Baked Cod with Olive Tapenade

Ingredients

- 4 cod fillets (about 6 oz each)
- 2 tablespoons olive oil
- 1 cup pitted Kalamata olives
- 1/4 cup sun-dried tomatoes, chopped
- 2 garlic cloves, minced
- 2 tablespoons capers, drained
- 2 tablespoons fresh parsley, chopped
- Juice of 1 lemon

Instructions

1. Preheat the oven to 375°F (190°C).
2. Place the cod fillets in a baking dish and brush with 1 tablespoon of olive oil.
3. In a food processor, combine the olives, sun-dried tomatoes, minced garlic, capers, parsley, remaining olive oil, and lemon juice. Pulse until finely chopped but not pureed.
4. Spread the olive tapenade evenly over the cod fillets.
5. Bake for 20-25 minutes, or until the fish is opaque and flakes easily with a fork.
6. Serve warm.

Nutrition Info (Per Serving)

- Calories: 280
- Protein: 32g
- Carbohydrates: 4g
- Fiber: 2g
- Sugars: 1g
- Fat: 15g

Servings: 4

Cooking Time: 25 minutes

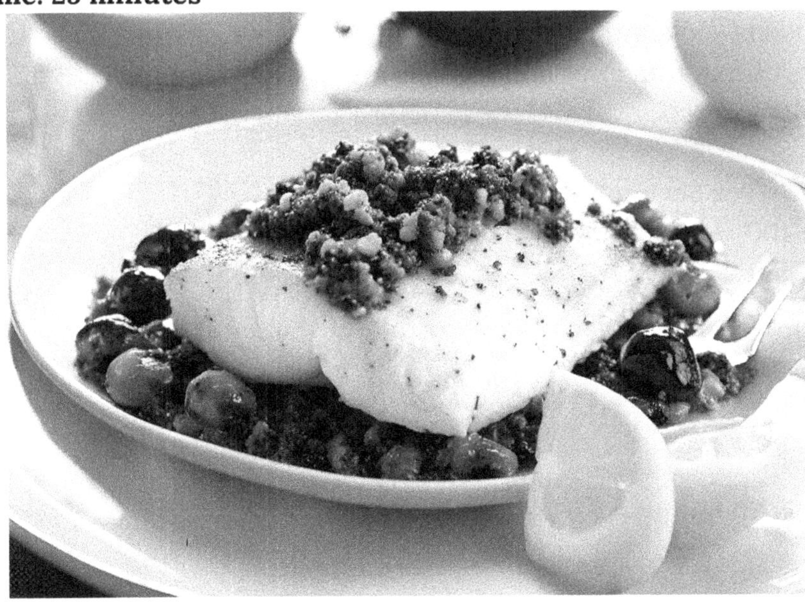

4. Seafood Paella with Brown Rice

Ingredients

- 1 lb shrimp, peeled and deveined
- 1 lb mussels, cleaned
- 1 lb calamari, cleaned and sliced
- 1 cup brown rice
- 4 cups low-sodium chicken broth
- 1 onion, chopped
- 1 red bell pepper, chopped
- 1 green bell pepper, chopped
- 3 garlic cloves, minced
- 1 teaspoon smoked paprika
- 1/2 teaspoon ground turmeric
- 1/2 teaspoon ground cumin
- 1 cup cherry tomatoes, halved
- 1/4 cup fresh parsley, chopped
- 2 tablespoons olive oil
- Juice of 1 lemon

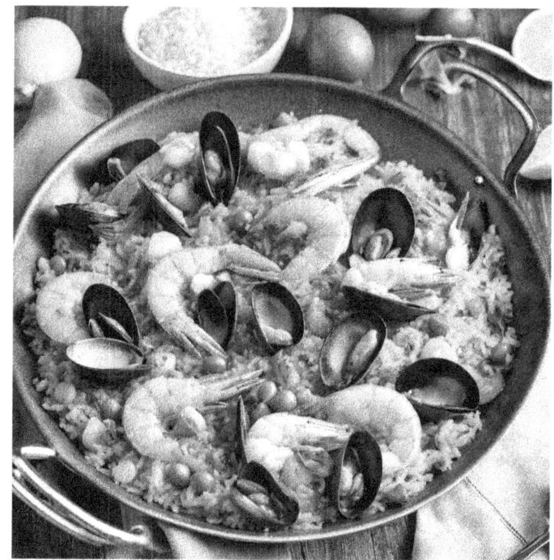

Instructions

1. In a large paella pan or skillet, heat the olive oil over medium heat. Add the onion, red bell pepper, and green bell pepper, and cook until softened, about 5 minutes.
2. Add the garlic, smoked paprika, turmeric, and cumin, and cook for another minute.
3. Stir in the brown rice and cook for 2-3 minutes until lightly toasted.
4. Pour in the chicken broth and bring to a boil. Reduce the heat to low, cover, and simmer for 30 minutes, or until the rice is tender.
5. Add the shrimp, mussels, and calamari, and cook for another 10 minutes, until the seafood is cooked through and the mussels have opened.
6. Stir in the cherry tomatoes and parsley, and cook for another 2-3 minutes.
7. Squeeze lemon juice over the paella before serving.
8. Serve warm.

Nutrition Info (Per Serving)

- Calories: 400
- Protein: 35g
- Carbohydrates: 40g
- Fiber: 4g
- Sugars: 4g
- Fat: 12g

Servings: 4

Cooking Time: 50 minutes

5. Asian-Style Steamed Snapper

Ingredients

- 4 snapper fillets (about 6 oz each)
- 2 tablespoons low-sodium soy sauce or tamari
- 1 tablespoon rice vinegar
- 1 tablespoon sesame oil
- 1 garlic clove, minced
- 1 tablespoon grated fresh ginger
- 2 green onions, thinly sliced
- 1 red chili, thinly sliced (optional)
- 1/4 cup fresh cilantro, chopped

Instructions

1. In a small bowl, mix the soy sauce, rice vinegar, sesame oil, minced garlic, and grated ginger.
2. Place the snapper fillets in a steamer basket and pour the soy sauce mixture over the fish.
3. Steam the fish over simmering water for 10-12 minutes, or until the fish is cooked through and flakes easily with a fork.
4. Transfer the snapper to a serving platter and garnish with green onions, red chili (if using), and cilantro.
5. Serve warm.

Nutrition Info (Per Serving)

- Calories: 220
- Protein: 30g
- Carbohydrates: 3g
- Fiber: 1g
- Sugars: 1g
- Fat: 9g

Servings: 4
Cooking Time: 15 minutes

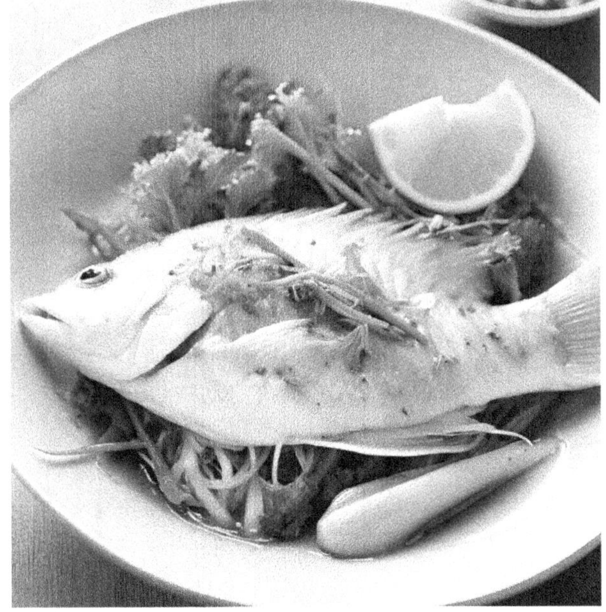

6. Lemon Garlic Butter Shrimp

Ingredients

- 1 lb shrimp, peeled and deveined
- 2 tablespoons olive oil
- 3 garlic cloves, minced
- Juice of 1 lemon
- 2 tablespoons fresh parsley, chopped
- 1 tablespoon butter

Instructions

1. Heat the olive oil in a large skillet over medium heat.
2. Add the garlic and cook for 1-2 minutes until fragrant.
3. Add the shrimp to the skillet and cook for 2-3 minutes on each side until pink and cooked through.
4. Stir in the lemon juice, parsley, and butter. Cook for an additional 1-2 minutes until the butter is melted and the shrimp are coated.
5. Serve warm.

Nutrition Info (Per Serving)

- Calories: 250
- Protein: 24g
- Carbohydrates: 4g
- Fiber: 1g
- Sugars: 0g
- Fat: 16g

Servings: 4
Cooking Time: 10 minutes

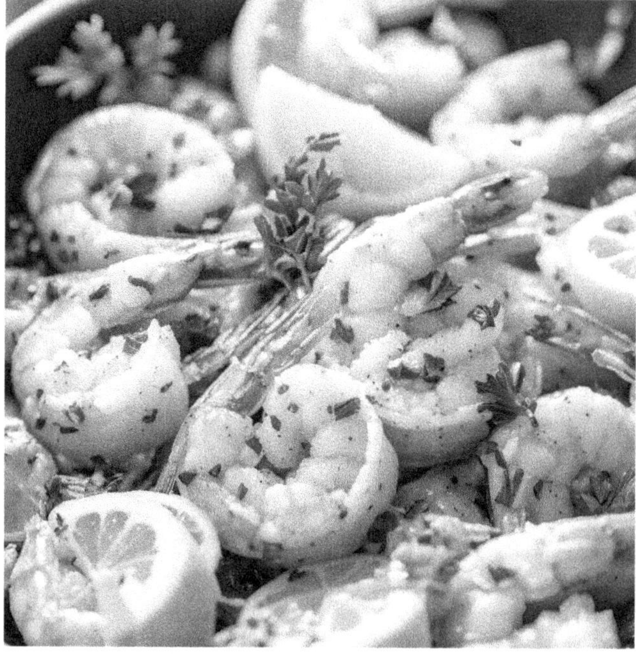

7. Herb-Crusted Tilapia with Steamed Vegetables

Ingredients

- 4 tilapia fillets
- 1/2 cup almond flour
- 1 tablespoon dried oregano
- 1 tablespoon dried basil
- 1 tablespoon dried thyme
- 2 tablespoons olive oil
- 1 lemon, sliced
- 2 cups broccoli florets
- 2 cups carrot slices
- 1 cup snap peas

Instructions

1. Preheat the oven to 375°F (190°C).
2. In a shallow dish, mix the almond flour, oregano, basil, and thyme.
3. Coat each tilapia fillet with the herb mixture.
4. Heat 1 tablespoon of olive oil in a large skillet over medium heat. Add the tilapia fillets and cook for 2-3 minutes on each side until golden brown.
5. Transfer the fillets to a baking sheet and top with lemon slices. Bake for 10-12 minutes until the fish is cooked through.
6. While the fish is baking, steam the broccoli, carrots, and snap peas until tender, about 5-7 minutes.
7. Drizzle the steamed vegetables with the remaining olive oil.
8. Serve the tilapia with the steamed vegetables.

Nutrition Info (Per Serving)

- Calories: 300
- Protein: 28g
- Carbohydrates: 12g
- Fiber: 5g
- Sugars: 4g
- Fat: 16g

Servings: 4
Cooking Time: 20 minutes

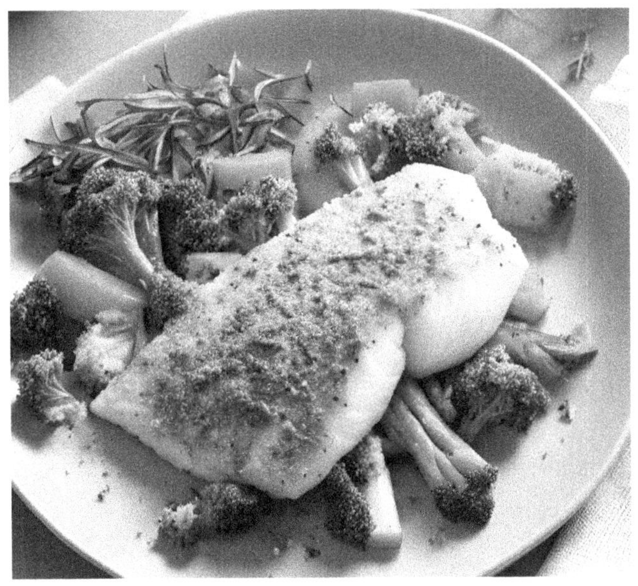

8. Spicy Grilled Mackerel

Ingredients

- 4 mackerel fillets
- 2 tablespoons olive oil
- 1 tablespoon smoked paprika
- 1 teaspoon ground cumin
- 1/2 teaspoon cayenne pepper
- 2 garlic cloves, minced
- Juice of 1 lime

Instructions

1. Preheat the grill to medium-high heat.
2. In a small bowl, mix the olive oil, smoked paprika, cumin, cayenne pepper, minced garlic, and lime juice.
3. Brush the mackerel fillets with the spice mixture.
4. Grill the mackerel fillets for 4-5 minutes on each side until cookcd through and the skin is crispy.
5. Serve warm.

Nutrition Info (Per Serving)

- Calories: 320
- Protein: 30g
- Carbohydrates: 2g
- Fiber: 1g
- Sugars: 0g
- Fat: 22g

Servings: 4
Cooking Time: 15 minutes

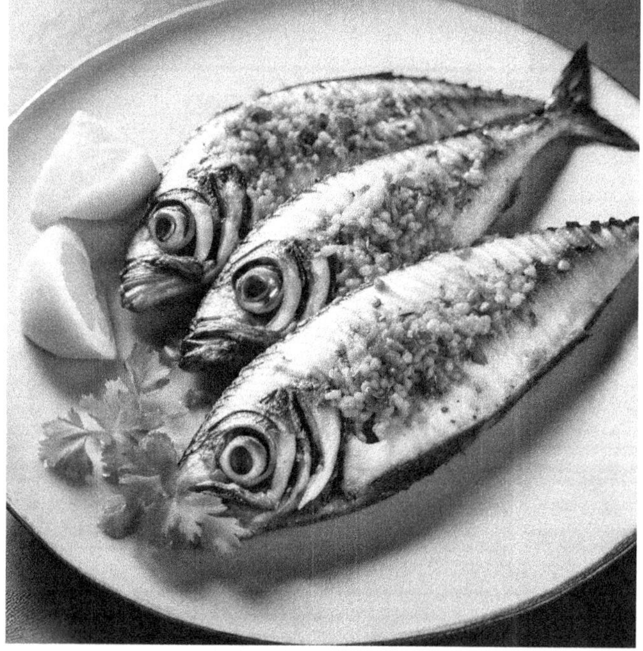

9. Clam Chowder with Sweet Potatoes

Ingredients

- 2 tablespoons olive oil
- 1 onion, chopped
- 3 garlic cloves, minced
- 2 large sweet potatoes, peeled and diced
- 3 cups low-sodium chicken broth
- 2 cups canned clams, with juice
- 1 cup unsweetened almond milk
- 1 teaspoon dried thyme
- 1/4 cup fresh parsley, chopped

Instructions

1. Heat the olive oil in a large pot over medium heat. Add the onion and garlic, and cook until softened, about 5 minutes.
2. Add the diced sweet potatoes and cook for another 5 minutes.
3. Pour in the chicken broth and bring to a boil. Reduce the heat and simmer for 15 minutes, or until the sweet potatoes are tender.
4. Add the clams with their juice, almond milk, and dried thyme. Simmer for another 5 minutes.
5. Stir in the fresh parsley.
6. Serve warm.

Nutrition Info (Per Serving)

- Calories: 250
- Protein: 15g
- Carbohydrates: 30g
- Fiber: 6g
- Sugars: 8g
- Fat: 8g

Servings: 4
Cooking Time: 30 minutes

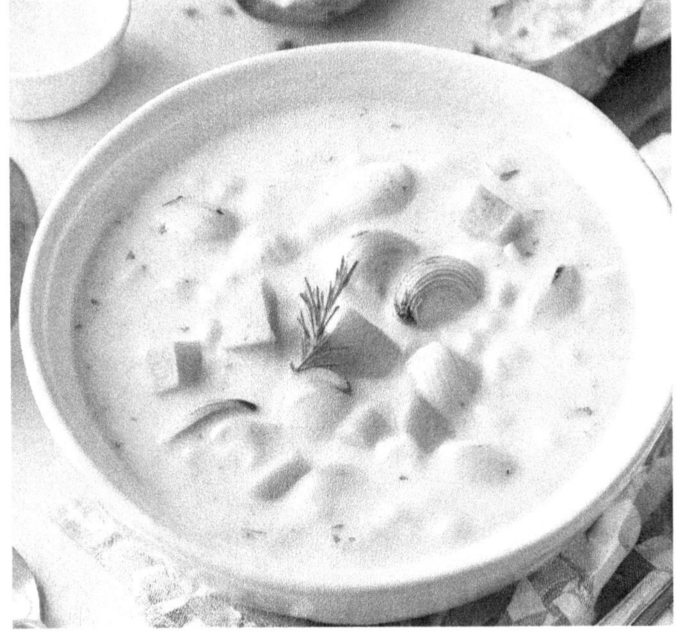

10. Grilled Trout with Parsley Salad
Ingredients

- 4 trout fillets
- 2 tablespoons olive oil
- Juice of 1 lemon
- 1 garlic clove, minced
- 1/4 cup fresh parsley, chopped
- 2 cups arugula
- 1/2 cup cherry tomatoes, halved
- 1/4 red onion, thinly sliced

Instructions

1. Preheat the grill to medium-high heat.
2. In a small bowl, mix 1 tablespoon of olive oil, lemon juice, minced garlic, and half of the chopped parsley.
3. Brush the trout fillets with the olive oil mixture.
4. Grill the trout fillets for 4-5 minutes on each side until cooked through and the skin is crispy.
5. In a large bowl, toss the arugula, cherry tomatoes, red onion, and remaining parsley with the remaining 1 tablespoon of olive oil.
6. Serve the grilled trout with the parsley salad.

Nutrition Info (Per Serving)

- Calories: 280
- Protein: 30g
- Carbohydrates: 5g
- Fiber: 2g
- Sugars: 2g
- Fat: 16g

Servings: 4
Cooking Time: 15 minutes

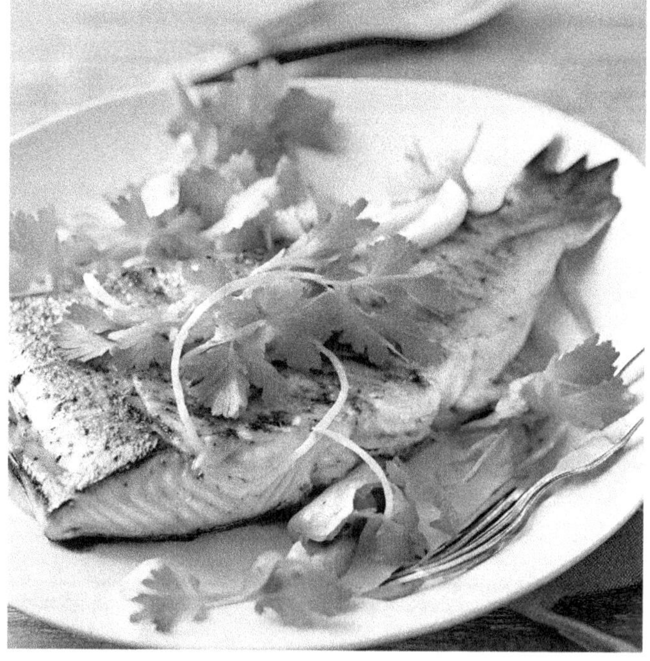

11. Salmon Poke Bowl

Ingredients

- 1 lb sushi-grade salmon, diced
- 2 tablespoons low-sodium soy sauce or tamari
- 1 tablespoon rice vinegar
- 1 tablespoon sesame oil
- 1 teaspoon grated fresh ginger
- 2 cups cooked brown rice
- 1 avocado, sliced
- 1 cup cucumber, julienned
- 1/2 cup shredded carrots
- 1/4 cup green onions, sliced
- 1 tablespoon sesame seeds

Instructions

1. In a medium bowl, mix the soy sauce, rice vinegar, sesame oil, and grated ginger.
2. Add the diced salmon to the bowl and toss to coat. Let it marinate for 10-15 minutes.
3. Divide the cooked brown rice among four bowls.
4. Top each bowl with the marinated salmon, avocado slices, cucumber, shredded carrots, and green onions.
5. Sprinkle with sesame seeds before serving.

Nutrition Info (Per Serving)

- Calories: 450
- Protein: 28g
- Carbohydrates: 38g
- Fiber: 6g
- Sugars: 3g
- Fat: 22g

Servings: 4

Cooking Time: 20 minutes

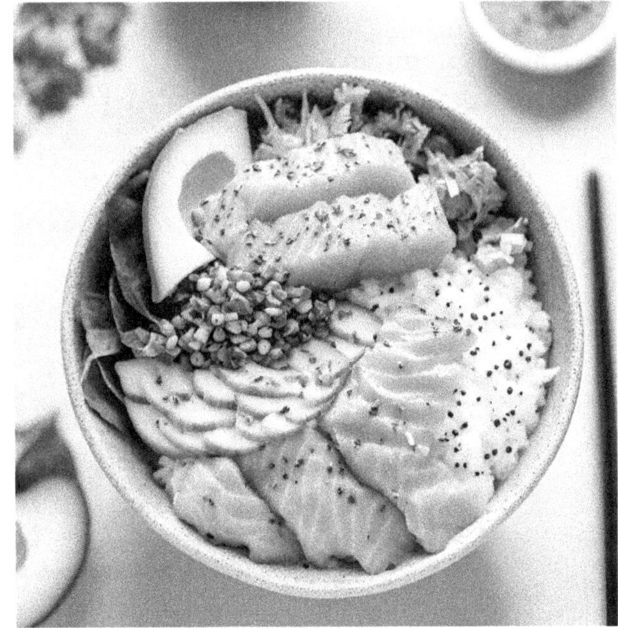

12. Baked Haddock with Tomato and Basil

Ingredients

- 4 haddock fillets
- 2 tablespoons olive oil
- 1 pint cherry tomatoes, halved
- 3 garlic cloves, minced
- 1/4 cup fresh basil, chopped
- Juice of 1 lemon

Instructions

1. Preheat the oven to 375°F (190°C).
2. Place the haddock fillets in a baking dish and brush with olive oil.
3. Top with cherry tomatoes, minced garlic, and lemon juice.
4. Bake for 20-25 minutes, or until the fish is cooked through and flakes easily with a fork.
5. Garnish with fresh basil before serving.
6. Serve warm.

Nutrition Info (Per Serving)

- Calories: 250
- Protein: 30g
- Carbohydrates: 6g
- Fiber: 2g
- Sugars: 3g
- Fat: 12g

Servings: 4
Cooking Time: 25 minutes

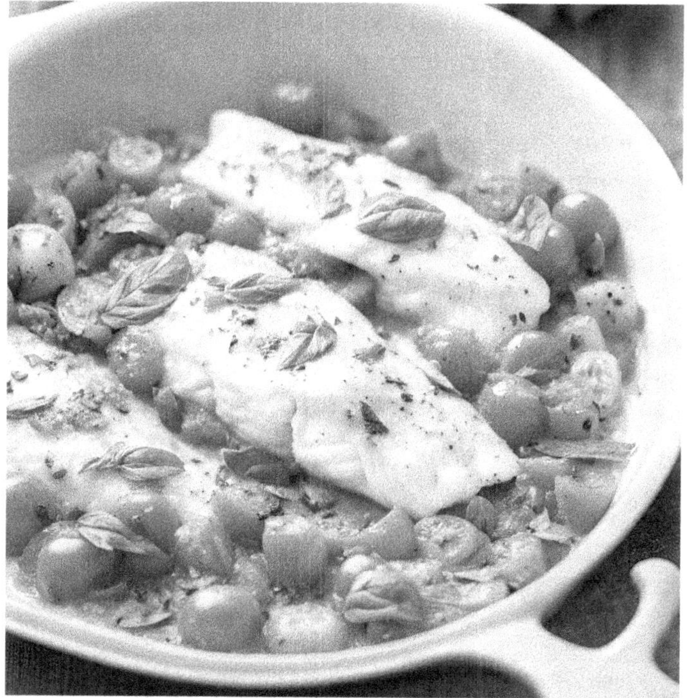

13. Fish Tacos with Cabbage Slaw

Ingredients

- 1 lb white fish fillets (such as cod or tilapia)
- 2 tablespoons olive oil
- 1 teaspoon ground cumin
- 1 teaspoon ground paprika
- 8 small corn tortillas
- 2 cups shredded cabbage
- 1/2 cup shredded carrots
- 1/4 cup fresh cilantro, chopped
- 1/4 cup Greek yogurt
- Juice of 1 lime

Instructions

1. Preheat the oven to 400°F (200°C).
2. Place the fish fillets on a baking sheet and brush with olive oil. Sprinkle with cumin and paprika.
3. Bake for 12-15 minutes, or until the fish is cooked through and flakes easily with a fork.
4. In a bowl, mix the shredded cabbage, carrots, cilantro, Greek yogurt, and lime juice to make the slaw.
5. Warm the tortillas in a dry skillet over medium heat.
6. Assemble the tacos by placing pieces of fish on each tortilla and topping with cabbage slaw.
7. Serve immediately.

Nutrition Info (Per Serving)

- Calories: 300
- Protein: 22g
- Carbohydrates: 32g
- Fiber: 6g
- Sugars: 4g
- Fat: 12g

Servings: 4

Cooking Time: 20 minutes

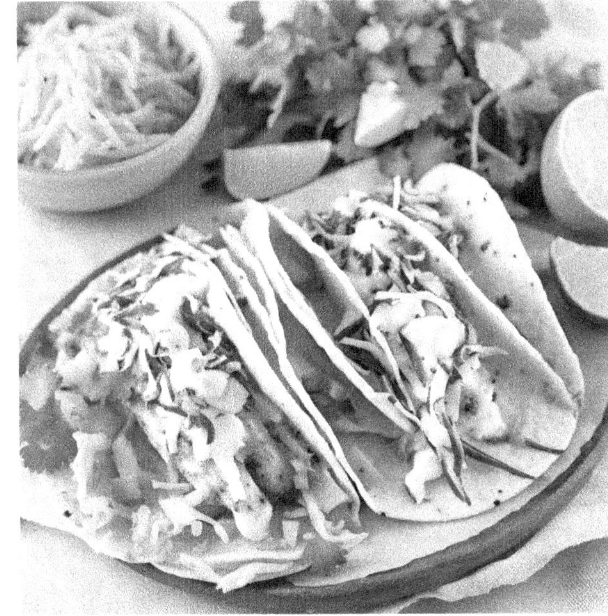

14. Prawn Risotto with Peas

Ingredients

- 1 lb prawns, peeled and deveined
- 1 cup Arborio rice
- 4 cups low-sodium chicken broth
- 1 cup frozen peas
- 1 small onion, finely chopped
- 2 garlic cloves, minced
- 1/2 cup dry white wine
- 2 tablespoons olive oil
- 1/4 cup grated Parmesan cheese
- 2 tablespoons fresh parsley, chopped

Instructions

1. In a medium saucepan, heat the chicken broth and keep it warm.
2. In a large skillet, heat the olive oil over medium heat. Add the onion and garlic, and cook until softened, about 5 minutes.
3. Add the Arborio rice and cook for 2-3 minutes, stirring constantly, until the rice is lightly toasted.
4. Pour in the white wine and cook until it is absorbed.
5. Add the warm chicken broth one ladle at a time, stirring frequently, until each addition is absorbed before adding the next. This process should take about 20 minutes.
6. When the rice is creamy and tender, stir in the prawns and peas. Cook for another 5-7 minutes until the prawns are cooked through.
7. Remove from heat and stir in the Parmesan cheese.
8. Garnish with fresh parsley and serve warm.

Nutrition Info (Per Serving)

- Calories: 350
- Protein: 25g
- Carbohydrates: 45g
- Fiber: 4g
- Sugars: 3g
- Fat: 10g

Servings: 4

Cooking Time: 30 minutes

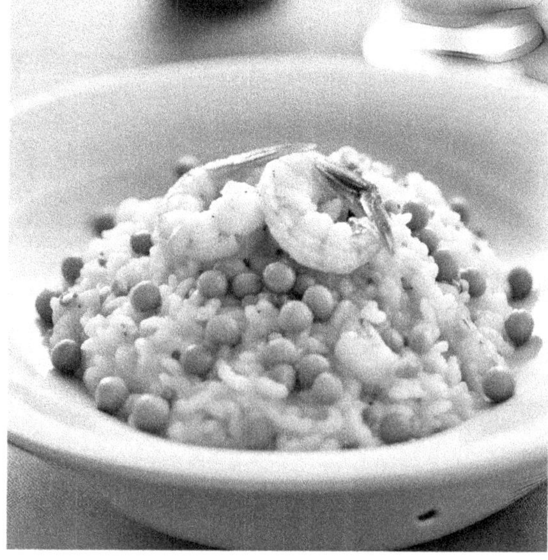

15. Lobster Salad with Mixed Greens

Ingredients

- 1 lb cooked lobster meat, chopped
- 4 cups mixed greens
- 1 avocado, diced
- 1/2 cup cherry tomatoes, halved
- 1/4 cup red onion, thinly sliced
- 2 tablespoons olive oil
- Juice of 1 lemon
- 1 tablespoon Dijon mustard

Instructions

1. In a large bowl, combine the mixed greens, avocado, cherry tomatoes, and red onion.
2. In a small bowl, whisk together the olive oil, lemon juice, and Dijon mustard.
3. Add the lobster meat to the mixed greens.
4. Drizzle the dressing over the salad and toss gently to combine.
5. Serve immediately.

Nutrition Info (Per Serving)

- Calories: 320
- Protein: 25g
- Carbohydrates: 12g
- Fiber: 6
- Sugars: 2g
- Fat: 20g

Servings: 4
Cooking Time: 15 minutes

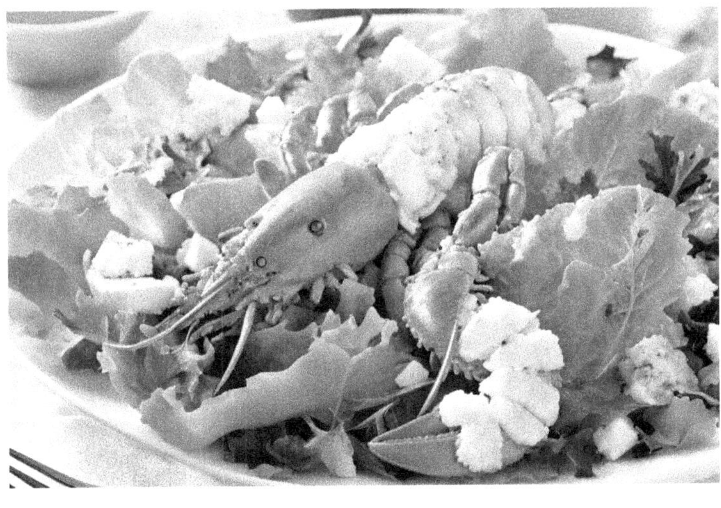

16. Anchovy and Tomato Pasta

Ingredients

- 8 oz gluten-free pasta
- 2 tablespoons olive oil
- 1 can (2 oz) anchovy fillets, drained and chopped
- 3 garlic cloves, minced
- 1 pint cherry tomatoes, halved
- 1/4 teaspoon red pepper flakes
- 1/4 cup fresh basil, chopped
- Juice of 1 lemon

Instructions

1. Cook the gluten-free pasta according to package instructions. Drain and set aside.
2. In a large skillet, heat the olive oil over medium heat. Add the minced garlic and cook for 1-2 minutes until fragrant.
3. Add the anchovy fillets and cook, stirring, until they dissolve into the oil.
4. Add the cherry tomatoes and red pepper flakes, and cook for 5-7 minutes until the tomatoes start to soften.
5. Stir in the cooked pasta and lemon juice. Toss to combine and heat through.
6. Garnish with fresh basil and serve warm.

Nutrition Info (Per Serving)

- Calories: 350
- Protein: 12g
- Carbohydrates: 45g
- Fiber: 4g
- Sugars: 5g
- Fat: 14g

Servings: 4
Cooking Time: 20 minutes

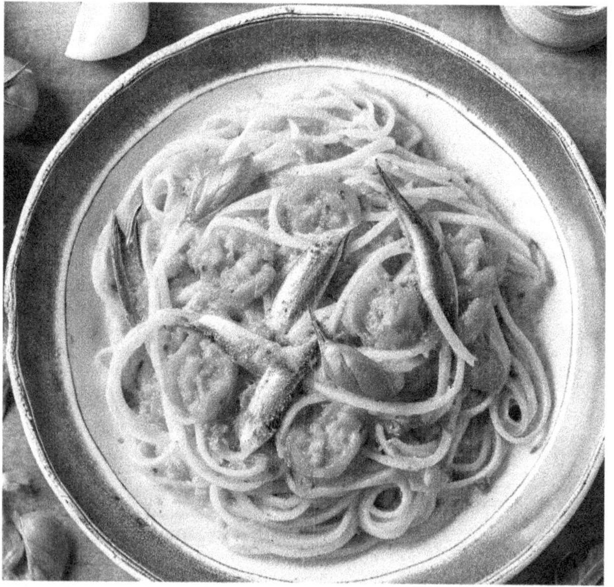

17. Pan-Seared Sardines with Lemon

Ingredients

- 8 fresh sardines, cleaned
- 2 tablespoons olive oil
- Juice of 1 lemon
- 2 garlic cloves, minced
- 1 tablespoon fresh parsley, chopped

Instructions

1. Heat the olive oil in a large skillet over medium-high heat.
2. Add the sardines to the skillet and cook for 3-4 minutes on each side, until golden brown and cooked through.
3. In a small bowl, mix the lemon juice and minced garlic.
4. Drizzle the lemon-garlic mixture over the sardines.
5. Garnish with fresh parsley and serve warm.

Nutrition Info (Per Serving)

- Calories: 250
- Protein: 20g
- Carbohydrates: 1g
- Fiber: 0g
- Sugars: 0g
- Fat: 18g

Servings: 4
Cooking Time: 10 minutes

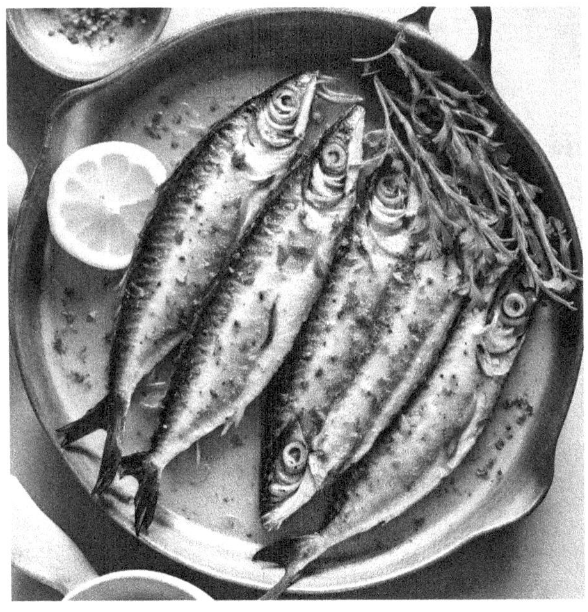

18. Oyster Stew
Ingredients

- 1 quart shucked oysters with their liquor
- 2 cups unsweetened almond milk
- 1 cup low-sodium chicken broth
- 2 tablespoons butter
- 1 small onion, finely chopped
- 2 celery stalks, finely chopped
- 1/4 teaspoon paprika
- 1 tablespoon fresh parsley, chopped

Instructions

1. In a large pot, melt the butter over medium heat. Add the onion and celery, and cook until softened, about 5 minutes.
2. Add the oysters with their liquor, almond milk, and chicken broth. Bring to a simmer.
3. Cook for about 5-7 minutes, until the edges of the oysters curl.
4. Stir in the paprika and parsley.
5. Serve warm.

Nutrition Info (Per Serving)

- Calories: 250
- Protein: 15g
- Carbohydrates: 10g
- Fiber: 2g
- Sugars: 3g
- Fat: 18g

Servings: 4
Cooking Time: 20 minutes

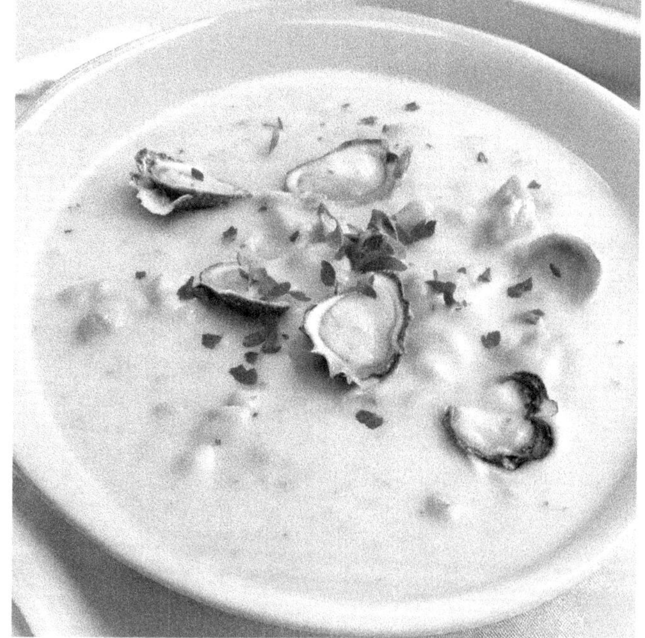

19. Catfish Amandine

Ingredients

- 4 catfish fillets
- 1/2 cup almond flour
- 2 tablespoons olive oil
- 1/4 cup sliced almonds
- Juice of 1 lemon
- 1 tablespoon fresh parsley, chopped

Instructions

1. Dredge the catfish fillets in almond flour, shaking off any excess.
2. Heat the olive oil in a large skillet over medium heat. Add the catfish fillets and cook for 4-5 minutes on each side, until golden brown and cooked through. Remove from the skillet and set aside.
3. In the same skillet, add the sliced almonds and cook until lightly toasted, about 2 minutes.
4. Add the lemon juice and parsley to the skillet, stirring to combine.
5. Pour the almond mixture over the catfish fillets.
6. Serve warm.

Nutrition Info (Per Serving)

- Calories: 300
- Protein: 28g
- Carbohydrates: 4g
- Fiber: 2g
- Sugars: 1g
- Fat: 20g

Servings: 4
Cooking Time: 15 minutes

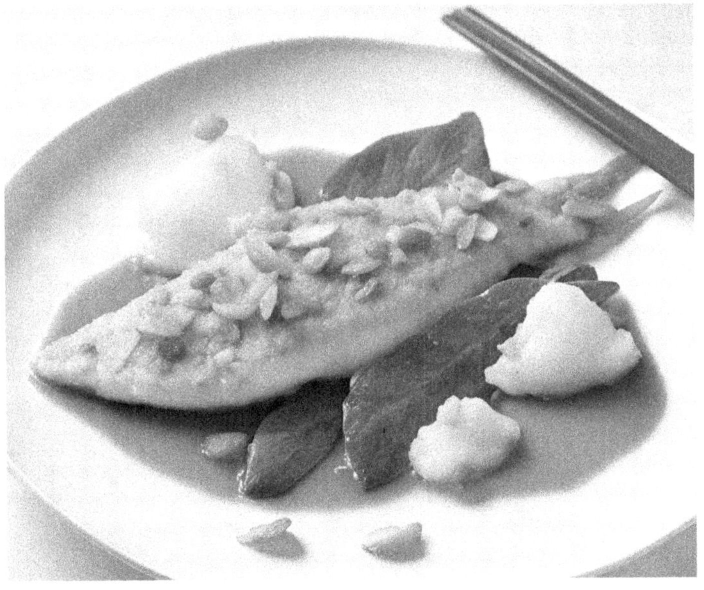

20. Octopus Salad with Citrus Dressing

Ingredients

- 1 lb cooked octopus, sliced
- 2 cups mixed greens
- 1 orange, segmented
- 1/2 red onion, thinly sliced
- 1/4 cup fresh cilantro, chopped
- 2 tablespoons olive oil
- Juice of 1 lemon
- Juice of 1 lime

Instructions

1. In a large bowl, combine the mixed greens, orange segments, red onion, and cilantro.
2. In a small bowl, whisk together the olive oil, lemon juice, and lime juice.
3. Add the sliced octopus to the salad and drizzle with the citrus dressing.
4. Toss gently to combine.
5. Serve immediately.

Nutrition Info (Per Serving)

- Calories: 250
- Protein: 20g
- Carbohydrates: 10g
- Fiber: 3g
- Sugars: 5g
- Fat: 14g

Servings: 4

Cooking Time: 15 minutes

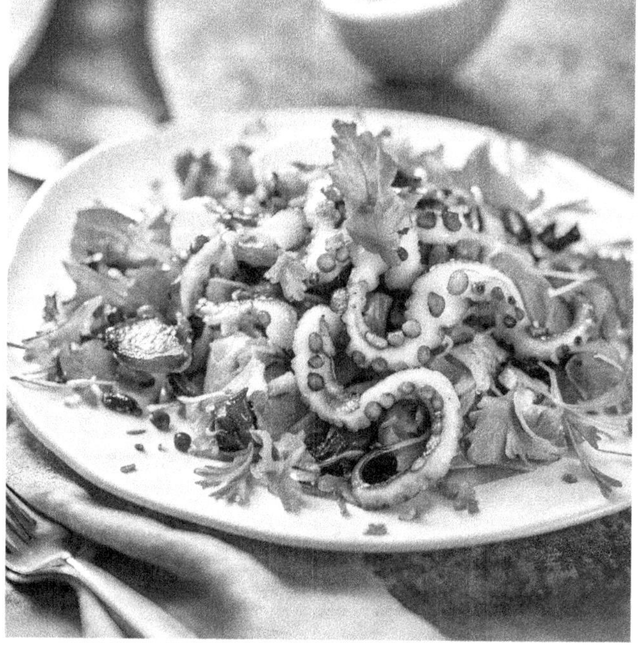

21. Steamed Scallops with Ginger and Soy

Ingredients

- 1 lb scallops
- 2 tablespoons low-sodium soy sauce or tamari
- 1 tablespoon rice vinegar
- 1 tablespoon sesame oil
- 1 tablespoon grated fresh ginger
- 2 green onions, thinly sliced

Instructions

1. In a small bowl, mix the soy sauce, rice vinegar, sesame oil, and grated ginger.
2. Place the scallops in a steamer basket over simmering water. Steam for 5-7 minutes, or until the scallops are opaque and cooked through.
3. Transfer the scallops to a serving dish and drizzle with the ginger soy sauce.
4. Garnish with green onions.
5. Serve warm.

Nutrition Info (Per Serving)

- Calories: 200
- Protein: 24g
- Carbohydrates: 3g
- Fiber: 1g
- Sugars: 1g
- Fat: 9g

Servings: 4
Cooking Time: 10 minutes

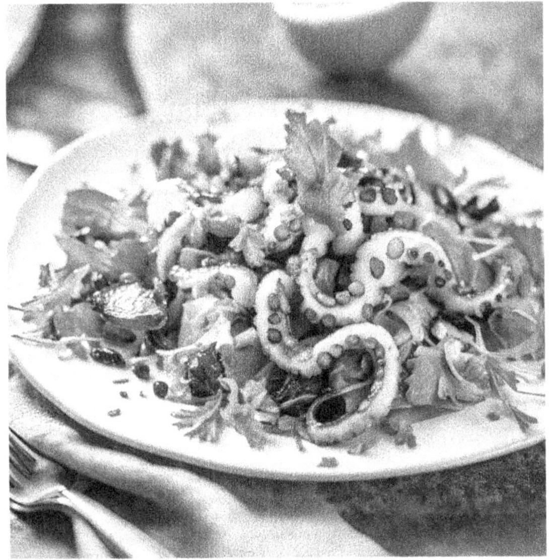

22. Shrimp Pad Thai

Ingredients

- 1 lb shrimp, peeled and deveined
- 8 oz rice noodles
- 2 tablespoons olive oil
- 2 garlic cloves, minced
- 2 eggs, lightly beaten
- 1 cup bean sprouts
- 1/4 cup peanuts, chopped
- 1/4 cup fresh cilantro, chopped
- 2 tablespoons low-sodium soy sauce or tamari
- 1 tablespoon rice vinegar
- 1 tablespoon lime juice
- 1 teaspoon honey

Instructions

1. Cook the rice noodles according to package instructions. Drain and set aside.
2. In a large skillet, heat the olive oil over medium heat. Add the garlic and cook for 1-2 minutes until fragrant.
3. Add the shrimp and cook for 3-4 minutes until pink and cooked through. Remove from the skillet and set aside.
4. Add the beaten eggs to the skillet and scramble until cooked through.
5. Return the shrimp to the skillet, along with the cooked noodles, bean sprouts, and chopped peanuts.
6. In a small bowl, mix the soy sauce, rice vinegar, lime juice, and honey. Pour the sauce over the noodle mixture and toss to combine.
7. Garnish with fresh cilantro before serving.
8. Serve warm.

Nutrition Info (Per Serving)

- Calories: 350
- Protein: 25g
- Carbohydrates: 40g
- Fiber: 3g
- Sugars: 5g
- Fat: 12g

Servings: 4
Cooking Time: 20 minutes

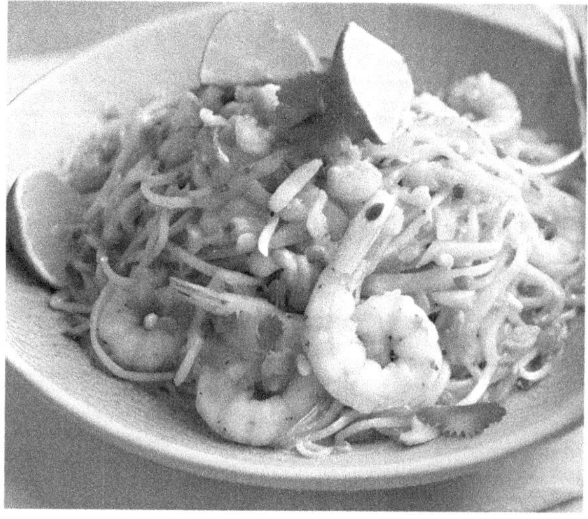

23. Cedar Plank Salmon with Rosemary

Ingredients

- 4 salmon fillets (about 6 oz each)
- 1 cedar plank, soaked in water for at least 1 hour
- 2 tablespoons olive oil
- 2 garlic cloves, minced
- 2 tablespoons fresh rosemary, chopped
- Juice of 1 lemon

Instructions

1. Preheat the grill to medium-high heat.
2. In a small bowl, mix the olive oil, minced garlic, rosemary, and lemon juice.
3. Brush the salmon fillets with the olive oil mixture.
4. Place the soaked cedar plank on the grill and heat for about 5 minutes.
5. Place the salmon fillets on the cedar plank and grill for 12-15 minutes, or until the salmon is cooked through and flakes easily with a fork.
6. Serve warm.

Nutrition Info (Per Serving)

- Calories: 350
- Protein: 34g
- Carbohydrates: 2g
- Fiber: 1g
- Sugars: 0g
- Fat: 22g

Servings: 4
Cooking Time: 20 minutes

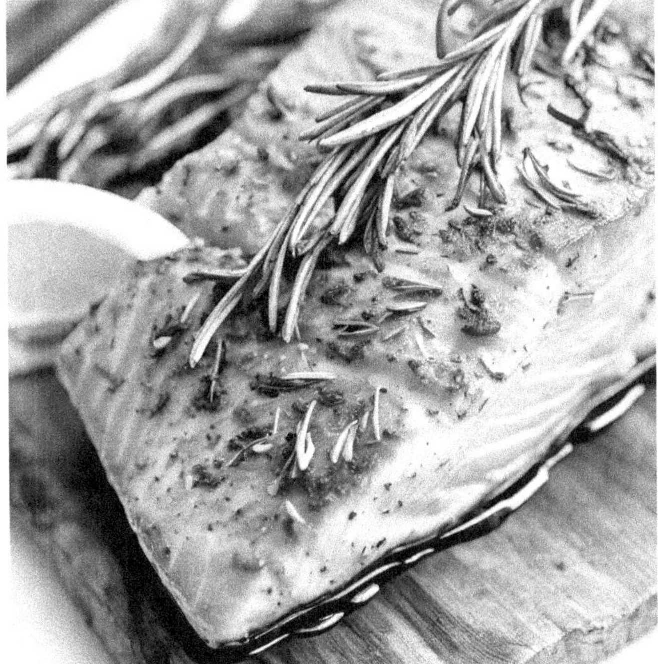

24. Sesame-Crusted Tuna Steaks

Ingredients

- 4 tuna steaks (about 6 oz each)
- 2 tablespoons olive oil
- 1/4 cup sesame seeds
- 2 tablespoons low-sodium soy sauce or tamari
- 1 tablespoon rice vinegar
- 1 tablespoon honey
- 1 tablespoon grated fresh ginger

Instructions

1. In a small bowl, mix the soy sauce, rice vinegar, honey, and grated ginger.
2. Brush the tuna steaks with the olive oil, then coat each steak with sesame seeds.
3. Heat a large skillet over medium-high heat. Add the tuna steaks and sear for 2-3 minutes on each side, until the sesame seeds are golden brown and the tuna is cooked to desired doneness.
4. Drizzle the soy sauce mixture over the tuna steaks before serving.
5. Serve warm.

Nutrition Info (Per Serving)

- Calories: 320
- Protein: 34g
- Carbohydrates: 5g
- Fiber: 1g
- Sugars: 2g
- Fat: 18g

Servings: 4
Cooking Time: 10 minutes

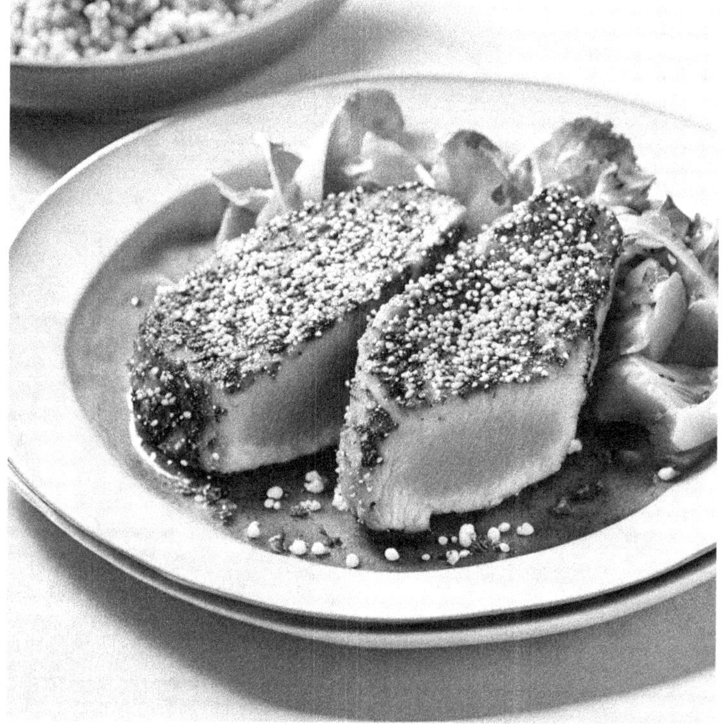

25. Sea Bass with Fennel and Orange

Ingredients

- 4 sea bass fillets
- 2 tablespoons olive oil
- 1 fennel bulb, thinly sliced
- 1 orange, peeled and segmented
- 2 garlic cloves, minced
- 1/4 cup fresh dill, chopped
- Juice of 1 lemon

Instructions

1. Preheat the oven to 375°F (190°C).
2. In a large oven-safe skillet, heat 1 tablespoon of olive oil over medium heat. Add the fennel and garlic, and cook until softened, about 5 minutes.
3. Add the orange segments and cook for another 2 minutes.
4. Push the fennel and orange to the sides of the skillet and add the sea bass fillets. Drizzle with the remaining olive oil and lemon juice.
5. Transfer the skillet to the oven and bake for 15-20 minutes, or until the fish is cooked through and flakes easily with a fork.
6. Garnish with fresh dill before serving.
7. Serve warm.

Nutrition Info (Per Serving)

- Calories: 300
- Protein: 28g
- Carbohydrates: 8g
- Fiber: 3g
- Sugars: 5g
- Fat: 18g

Servings: 4
Cooking Time: 25 minutes

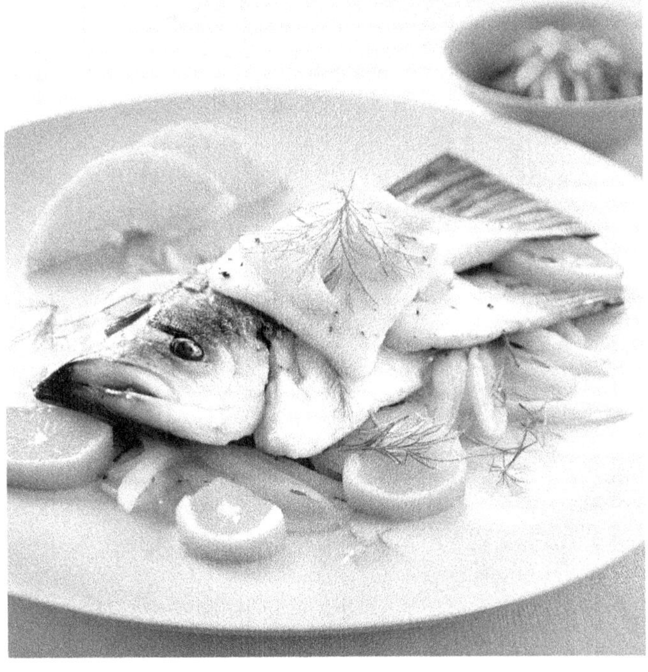

Soup and Stew Recipes

1. Chicken Bone Broth

Ingredients

- 2 lbs chicken bones (preferably with some meat on them)
- 2 tablespoons apple cider vinegar
- 1 onion, quartered
- 2 carrots, chopped
- 2 celery stalks, chopped
- 3 garlic cloves, smashed
- 1 tablespoon fresh thyme
- 1 tablespoon fresh rosemary
- 8 cups water

Instructions

1. Place the chicken bones in a large pot or slow cooker.
2. Add the apple cider vinegar and enough water to cover the bones. Let it sit for 30 minutes.
3. Add the onion, carrots, celery, garlic, thyme, and rosemary.
4. Pour in the remaining water.
5. Bring to a boil, then reduce the heat and simmer for 12-24 hours. If using a slow cooker, cook on low for the same amount of time.
6. Strain the broth through a fine mesh sieve, discarding the solids.
7. Let the broth cool and refrigerate. Skim off the fat that solidifies on the top before using.
8. Serve warm.

Nutrition Info (Per Serving)

- Calories: 50
- Protein: 10g
- Carbohydrates: 2g
- Fiber: 1g
- Sugars: 1g
- Fat: 1g

Servings: 8
Cooking Time: 12-24 hours

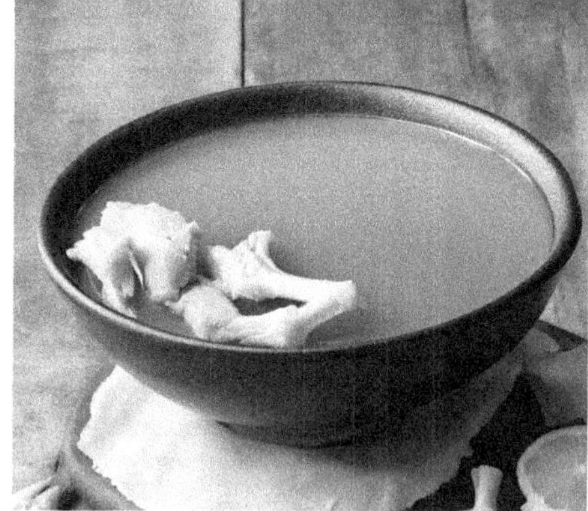

2. Turmeric Lentil Stew

Ingredients

- 1 cup red lentils, rinsed
- 2 tablespoons olive oil
- 1 onion, chopped
- 3 garlic cloves, minced
- 1 tablespoon grated fresh ginger
- 1 tablespoon ground turmeric
- 1 teaspoon ground cumin
- 1 teaspoon ground coriander
- 4 cups low-sodium vegetable broth
- 2 carrots, chopped
- 2 celery stalks, chopped
- 1 can (14.5 oz) diced tomatoes
- 1 cup baby spinach
- Juice of 1 lemon

Instructions

1. In a large pot, heat the olive oil over medium heat. Add the onion, garlic, and ginger, and cook until softened, about 5 minutes.
2. Stir in the turmeric, cumin, and coriander, and cook for another minute.
3. Add the lentils, vegetable broth, carrots, celery, and diced tomatoes.
4. Bring to a boil, then reduce the heat and simmer for 25-30 minutes, or until the lentils and vegetables are tender.
5. Stir in the baby spinach and lemon juice, and cook for another 2-3 minutes until the spinach is wilted.
6. Serve warm.

Nutrition Info (Per Serving)

- Calories: 250
- Protein: 12g
- Carbohydrates: 40g
- Fiber: 15g
- Sugars: 8g
- Fat: 7g

Servings: 4
Cooking Time: 40 minutes

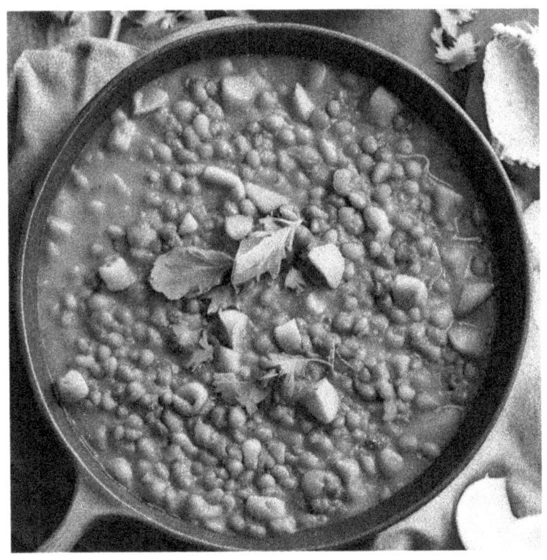

3. Sweet Potato and Roasted Red Pepper Soup

Ingredients

- 2 tablespoons olive oil
- 1 onion, chopped
- 3 garlic cloves, minced
- 2 large sweet potatoes, peeled and chopped
- 2 roasted red peppers, chopped
- 4 cups low-sodium vegetable broth
- 1 teaspoon smoked paprika
- 1/2 teaspoon ground cumin
- 1/2 cup coconut milk
- 1/4 cup fresh cilantro, chopped (for garnish)

Instructions

1. In a large pot, heat the olive oil over medium heat. Add the onion and garlic, and cook until softened, about 5 minutes.
2. Add the sweet potatoes, roasted red peppers, vegetable broth, smoked paprika, and cumin.
3. Bring to a boil, then reduce the heat and simmer for 20-25 minutes, or until the sweet potatoes are tender.
4. Use an immersion blender to puree the soup until smooth, or transfer the soup to a blender and blend in batches.
5. Stir in the coconut milk and heat through.
6. Garnish with fresh cilantro and serve warm.

Nutrition Info (Per Serving)

- Calories: 220
- Protein: 4g
- Carbohydrates: 35g
- Fiber: 6g
- Sugars: 10g
- Fat: 9g

Servings: 4

Cooking Time: 30 minutes

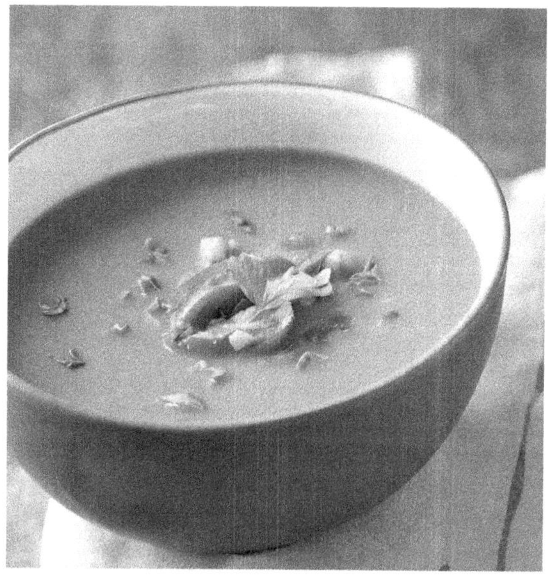

4. Miso Soup with Tofu and Seaweed

Ingredients

- 4 cups water
- 2 tablespoons miso paste
- 1 cup tofu, cubed
- 1/4 cup dried wakame seaweed
- 1/4 cup green onions, sliced
- 1 tablespoon grated fresh ginger

Instructions

1. In a large pot, bring the water to a simmer.
2. Add the miso paste and whisk until fully dissolved.
3. Stir in the tofu, wakame seaweed, and grated ginger.
4. Simmer for 5-7 minutes, until the tofu is heated through and the seaweed is rehydrated.
5. Garnish with green onions.
6. Serve warm.

Nutrition Info (Per Serving)

- Calories: 80
- Protein: 6g
- Carbohydrates: 6g
- Fiber: 1g
- Sugars: 1g
- Fat: 4g

Servings: 4
Cooking Time: 10 minutes

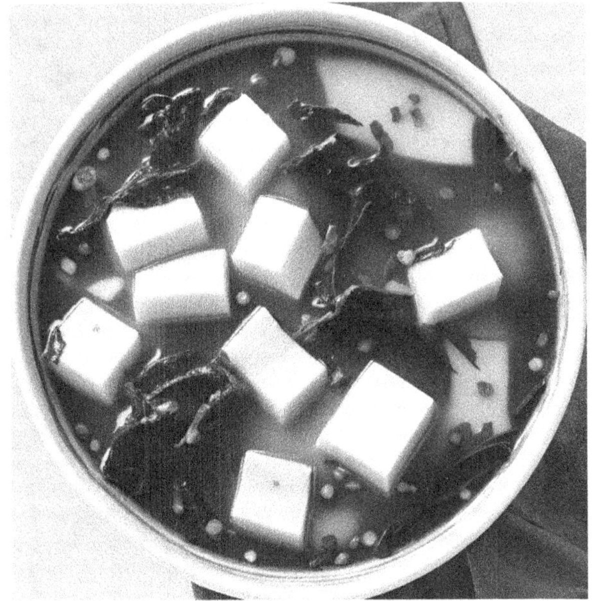

5. Beetroot and Ginger Soup

Ingredients

- 2 tablespoons olive oil
- 1 onion, chopped
- 3 garlic cloves, minced
- 1 tablespoon grated fresh ginger
- 4 large beetroots, peeled and chopped
- 4 cups low-sodium vegetable broth
- 1 apple, peeled, cored, and chopped
- Juice of 1 lemon
- 1/4 cup fresh dill, chopped (for garnish)

Instructions

1. In a large pot, heat the olive oil over medium heat. Add the onion, garlic, and ginger, and cook until softened, about 5 minutes.
2. Add the chopped beetroots, vegetable broth, and apple.
3. Bring to a boil, then reduce the heat and simmer for 25-30 minutes, or until the beetroots are tender.
4. Use an immersion blender to puree the soup until smooth, or transfer the soup to a blender and blend in batches.
5. Stir in the lemon juice and heat through.
6. Garnish with fresh dill and serve warm.

Nutrition Info (Per Serving)

- Calories: 150
- Protein: 3g
- Carbohydrates: 26g
- Fiber: 6g
- Sugars: 15g
- Fat: 5g

Servings: 4
Cooking Time: 35 minutes

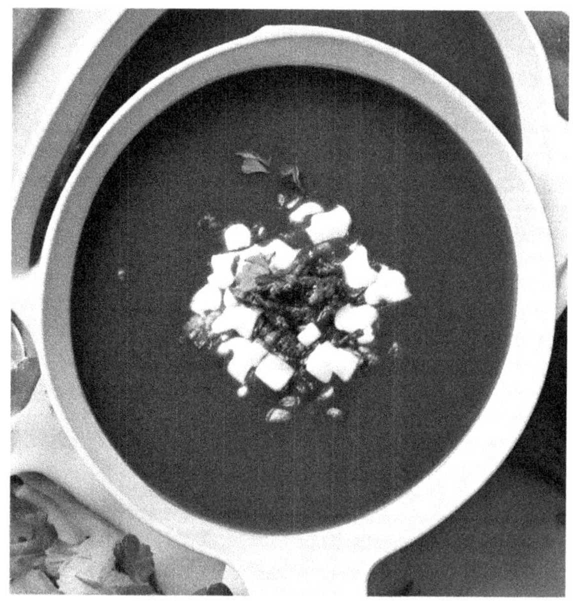

6. Split Pea Soup with Ham

Ingredients

- 1 lb dried split peas, rinsed
- 1 lb ham hock or diced ham
- 1 onion, chopped
- 2 carrots, chopped
- 2 celery stalks, chopped
- 3 garlic cloves, minced
- 1 teaspoon dried thyme
- 1 bay leaf
- 6 cups low-sodium chicken broth
- 2 cups water
- 1 tablespoon olive oil

Instructions

1. In a large pot, heat the olive oil over medium heat. Add the onion, garlic, carrots, and celery. Cook until softened, about 5 minutes.
2. Add the split peas, ham hock or diced ham, thyme, and bay leaf. Stir to combine.
3. Pour in the chicken broth and water. Bring to a boil, then reduce the heat and simmer for 1.5 to 2 hours, or until the peas are tender and the soup is thickened.
4. Remove the ham hock, shred the meat, and return it to the pot. Discard the bay leaf.
5. Serve warm.

Nutrition Info (Per Serving)

- Calories: 300
- Protein: 20g
- Carbohydrates: 40g
- Fiber: 16g
- Sugars: 6g
- Fat: 8g

Servings: 6

Cooking Time: 2 hours

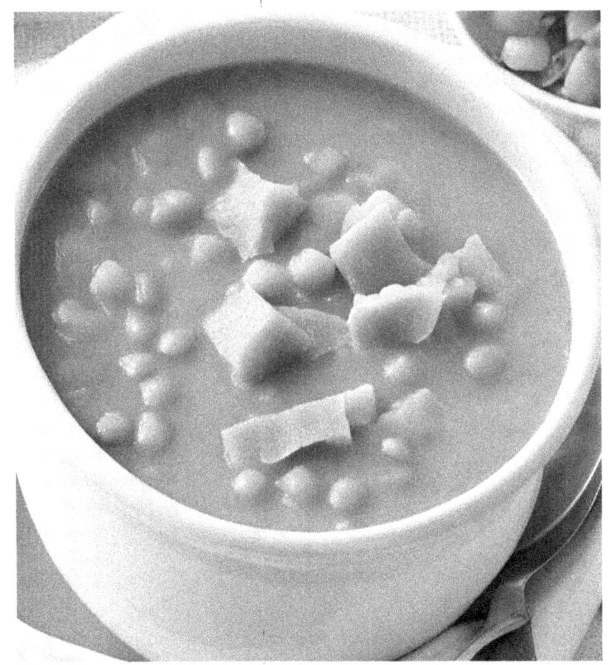

7. Pumpkin Soup with Nutmeg

Ingredients

- 2 tablespoons olive oil
- 1 onion, chopped
- 3 garlic cloves, minced
- 4 cups pumpkin puree
- 4 cups low-sodium vegetable broth
- 1 cup unsweetened almond milk
- 1/2 teaspoon ground nutmeg
- 1/2 teaspoon ground cinnamon
- 1/4 teaspoon ground ginger

Instructions

1. In a large pot, heat the olive oil over medium heat. Add the onion and garlic, and cook until softened, about 5 minutes.
2. Add the pumpkin puree, vegetable broth, almond milk, nutmeg, cinnamon, and ginger. Stir to combine.
3. Bring to a boil, then reduce the heat and simmer for 20 minutes, stirring occasionally.
4. Use an immersion blender to puree the soup until smooth, or transfer the soup to a blender and blend in batches.
5. Serve warm.

Nutrition Info (Per Serving)

- Calories: 150
- Protein: 3g
- Carbohydrates: 24g
- Fiber: 6g
- Sugars: 10g
- Fat: 5g

Servings: 4
Cooking Time: 30 minutes

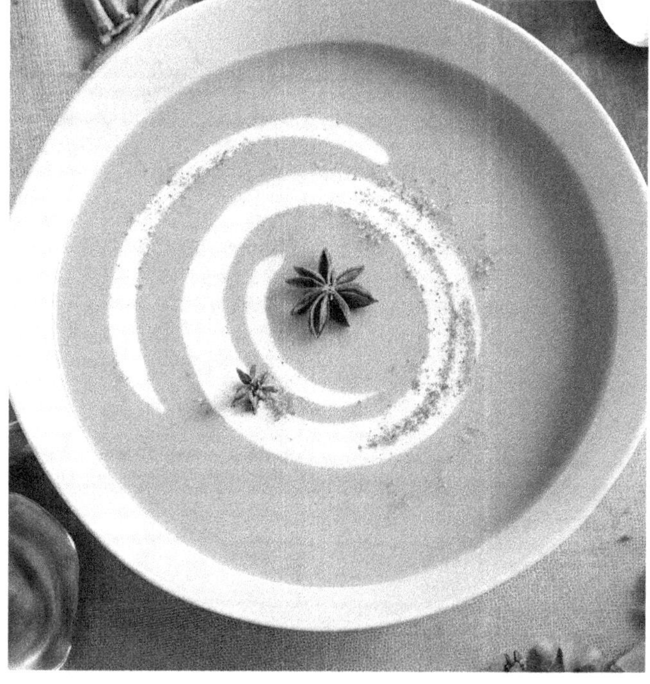

8. Kale and White Bean Soup

Ingredients

- 2 tablespoons olive oil
- 1 onion, chopped
- 3 garlic cloves, minced
- 4 cups chopped kale
- 2 cans (14.5 oz each) white beans, drained and rinsed
- 4 cups low-sodium vegetable broth
- 1 teaspoon dried thyme
- 1 teaspoon dried rosemary
- Juice of 1 lemon

Instructions

1. In a large pot, heat the olive oil over medium heat. Add the onion and garlic, and cook until softened, about 5 minutes.
2. Add the kale and cook until wilted, about 3 minutes.
3. Stir in the white beans, vegetable broth, thyme, and rosemary. Bring to a boil, then reduce the heat and simmer for 20 minutes.
4. Stir in the lemon juice.
5. Serve warm.

Nutrition Info (Per Serving)

- Calories: 200
- Protein: 10g
- Carbohydrates: 30g
- Fiber: 10g
- Sugars: 4g
- Fat: 6g

Servings: 4
Cooking Time: 30 minutes

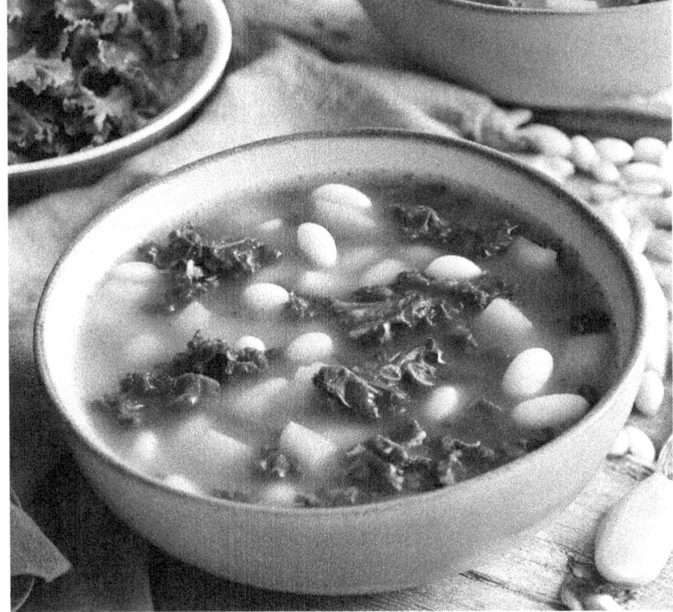

9. Tomato Basil Soup

Ingredients

- 2 tablespoons olive oil
- 1 onion, chopped
- 3 garlic cloves, minced
- 2 cans (28 oz each) diced tomatoes
- 4 cups low-sodium vegetable broth
- 1/2 cup fresh basil leaves, chopped
- 1 teaspoon dried oregano
- 1/2 cup unsweetened almond milk

Instructions

1. In a large pot, heat the olive oil over medium heat. Add the onion and garlic, and cook until softened, about 5 minutes.
2. Add the diced tomatoes, vegetable broth, basil, and oregano. Bring to a boil, then reduce the heat and simmer for 20 minutes.
3. Use an immersion blender to puree the soup until smooth, or transfer the soup to a blender and blend in batches.
4. Stir in the almond milk and heat through.
5. Serve warm.

Nutrition Info (Per Serving)

- Calories: 140
- Protein: 3g
- Carbohydrates: 18g
- Fiber: 4g
- Sugars: 10g
- Fat: 6g

Servings: 4

Cooking Time: 30 minutes

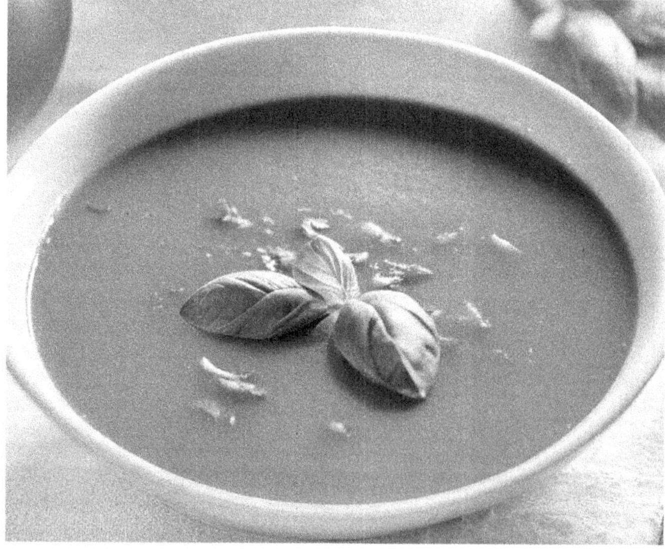

10. Vegetable Minestrone

Ingredients

- 2 tablespoons olive oil
- 1 onion, chopped
- 3 garlic cloves, minced
- 2 carrots, chopped
- 2 celery stalks, chopped
- 1 zucchini, chopped
- 1 can (14.5 oz) diced tomatoes
- 4 cups low-sodium vegetable broth
- 1 cup cooked cannellini beans
- 1 cup cooked kidney beans
- 1 cup gluten-free pasta
- 1 teaspoon dried basil
- 1 teaspoon dried oregano
- 1/2 cup fresh spinach, chopped

Instructions

1. In a large pot, heat the olive oil over medium heat. Add the onion, garlic, carrots, and celery, and cook until softened, about 5 minutes.
2. Add the zucchini, diced tomatoes, vegetable broth, cannellini beans, kidney beans, basil, and oregano. Bring to a boil.
3. Add the gluten-free pasta and cook for 10 minutes, or until the pasta is tender.
4. Stir in the fresh spinach and cook for another 2-3 minutes until wilted.
5. Serve warm.

Nutrition Info (Per Serving)

- Calories: 250
- Protein: 8g
- Carbohydrates: 40g
- Fiber: 8g
- Sugars: 10g
- Fat: 7g

Servings: 6
Cooking Time: 30 minutes

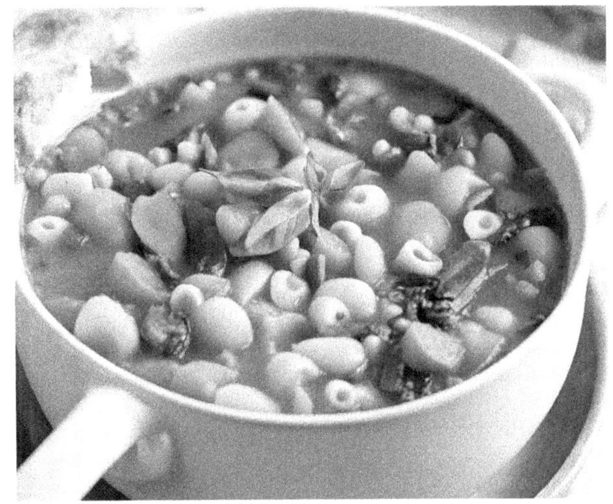

11. Moroccan Spiced Chickpea Soup

Ingredients

- 2 tablespoons olive oil
- 1 onion, chopped
- 3 garlic cloves, minced
- 1 tablespoon grated fresh ginger
- 1 teaspoon ground cumin
- 1 teaspoon ground coriander
- 1 teaspoon ground cinnamon
- 1/2 teaspoon ground turmeric
- 1/4 teaspoon ground cayenne pepper
- 1 can (14.5 oz) diced tomatoes
- 4 cups low-sodium vegetable broth
- 2 cans (14.5 oz each) chickpeas, drained and rinsed
- 1/4 cup fresh cilantro, chopped (for garnish)

Instructions

1. In a large pot, heat the olive oil over medium heat. Add the onion, garlic, and ginger, and cook until softened, about 5 minutes.
2. Stir in the cumin, coriander, cinnamon, turmeric, and cayenne pepper, and cook for another minute.
3. Add the diced tomatoes, vegetable broth, and chickpeas. Bring to a boil, then reduce the heat and simmer for 20 minutes.
4. Use an immersion blender to puree the soup slightly, leaving some chunks for texture, or transfer half of the soup to a blender and blend until smooth, then return to the pot.
5. Garnish with fresh cilantro before serving.
6. Serve warm.

Nutrition Info (Per Serving)

- Calories: 220
- Protein: 8g
- Carbohydrates: 34g
- Fiber: 10g
- Sugars: 8g
- Fat: 7g

Servings: 4
Cooking Time: 30 minutes

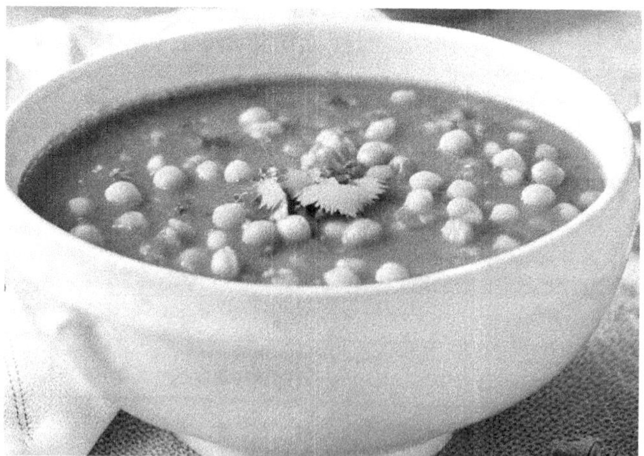

12. Mushroom and Barley Soup

Ingredients

- 2 tablespoons olive oil
- 1 onion, chopped
- 3 garlic cloves, minced
- 2 cups sliced mushrooms (cremini, shiitake, or button)
- 1 carrot, chopped
- 2 celery stalks, chopped
- 3/4 cup pearl barley
- 6 cups low-sodium vegetable broth
- 1 teaspoon dried thyme
- 1 bay leaf
- 1/4 cup fresh parsley, chopped

Instructions

1. In a large pot, heat the olive oil over medium heat. Add the onion and garlic, and cook until softened, about 5 minutes.
2. Add the mushrooms, carrot, and celery, and cook for another 5 minutes.
3. Stir in the barley, vegetable broth, thyme, and bay leaf. Bring to a boil, then reduce the heat and simmer for 45-50 minutes, or until the barley is tender.
4. Remove the bay leaf and stir in the fresh parsley.
5. Serve warm.

Nutrition Info (Per Serving)

- Calories: 200
- Protein: 6g
- Carbohydrates: 34g
- Fiber: 7g
- Sugars: 6g
- Fat: 6g

Servings: 6
Cooking Time: 60 minutes

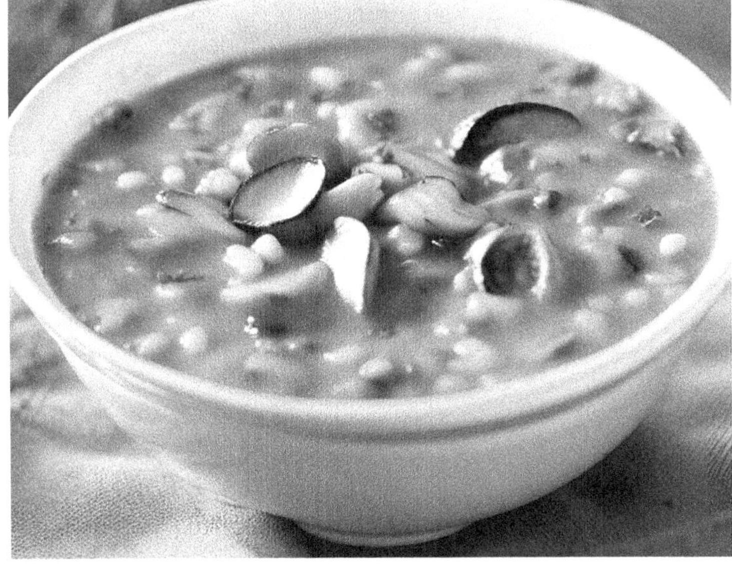

13. Thai Coconut Shrimp Soup

Ingredients

- 1 lb shrimp, peeled and deveined
- 2 tablespoons olive oil
- 1 onion, chopped
- 3 garlic cloves, minced
- 1 tablespoon grated fresh ginger
- 2 cups sliced mushrooms
- 1 red bell pepper, chopped
- 4 cups low-sodium chicken broth
- 1 can (14 oz) coconut milk
- 2 tablespoons red curry paste
- 1 tablespoon fish sauce
- 1 lime, juiced
- 1/4 cup fresh cilantro, chopped

Instructions

1. In a large pot, heat the olive oil over medium heat. Add the onion, garlic, and ginger, and cook until softened, about 5 minutes.
2. Add the mushrooms and red bell pepper, and cook for another 5 minutes.
3. Stir in the chicken broth, coconut milk, red curry paste, and fish sauce. Bring to a simmer.
4. Add the shrimp and cook for 5-7 minutes, until the shrimp are cooked through.
5. Stir in the lime juice and garnish with fresh cilantro.
6. Serve warm.

Nutrition Info (Per Serving)

- Calories: 300
- Protein: 22g
- Carbohydrates: 10g
- Fiber: 2g
- Sugars: 4g
- Fat: 20g

Servings: 4

Cooking Time: 30 minutes

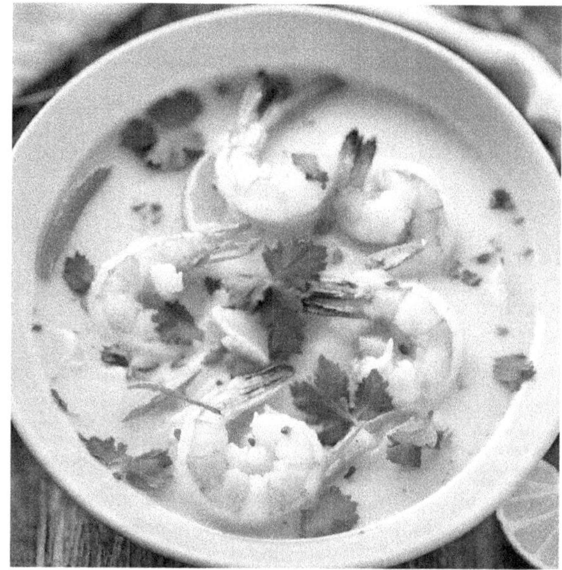

14. Italian Lentil Soup

Ingredients

- 2 tablespoons olive oil
- 1 onion, chopped
- 3 garlic cloves, minced
- 2 carrots, chopped
- 2 celery stalks, chopped
- 1 cup dried lentils, rinsed
- 1 can (14.5 oz) diced tomatoes
- 4 cups low-sodium vegetable broth
- 1 teaspoon dried basil
- 1 teaspoon dried oregano
- 1/4 teaspoon red pepper flakes
- 1/4 cup fresh parsley, chopped

Instructions

1. In a large pot, heat the olive oil over medium heat. Add the onion, garlic, carrots, and celery, and cook until softened, about 5 minutes.
2. Stir in the lentils, diced tomatoes, vegetable broth, basil, oregano, and red pepper flakes. Bring to a boil, then reduce the heat and simmer for 30-35 minutes, or until the lentils are tender.
3. Stir in the fresh parsley.
4. Serve warm.

Nutrition Info (Per Serving)

- Calories: 250
- Protein: 12g
- Carbohydrates: 40g
- Fiber: 15g
- Sugars: 8g
- Fat: 7g

Servings: 4
Cooking Time: 40 minutes

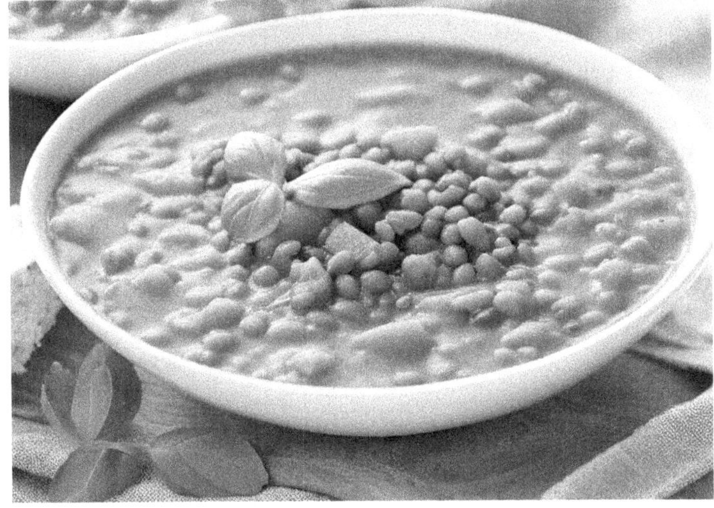

15. Spicy Black Bean Soup

Ingredients

- 2 tablespoons olive oil
- 1 onion, chopped
- 3 garlic cloves, minced
- 1 bell pepper, chopped
- 1 jalapeño, seeded and chopped
- 2 cans (14.5 oz each) black beans, drained and rinsed
- 4 cups low-sodium vegetable broth
- 1 teaspoon ground cumin
- 1 teaspoon smoked paprika
- 1/2 teaspoon ground coriander
- Juice of 1 lime
- 1/4 cup fresh cilantro, chopped

Instructions

1. In a large pot, heat the olive oil over medium heat. Add the onion, garlic, bell pepper, and jalapeño, and cook until softened, about 5 minutes.
2. Stir in the black beans, vegetable broth, cumin, smoked paprika, and coriander. Bring to a boil, then reduce the heat and simmer for 20-25 minutes.
3. Use an immersion blender to puree the soup slightly, leaving some chunks for texture, or transfer half of the soup to a blender and blend until smooth, then return to the pot.
4. Stir in the lime juice and garnish with fresh cilantro.
5. Serve warm.

Nutrition Info (Per Serving)

- Calories: 220
- Protein: 10g
- Carbohydrates: 35g
- Fiber: 12g
- Sugars: 5g
- Fat: 6g

Servings: 4
Cooking Time: 30 minutes

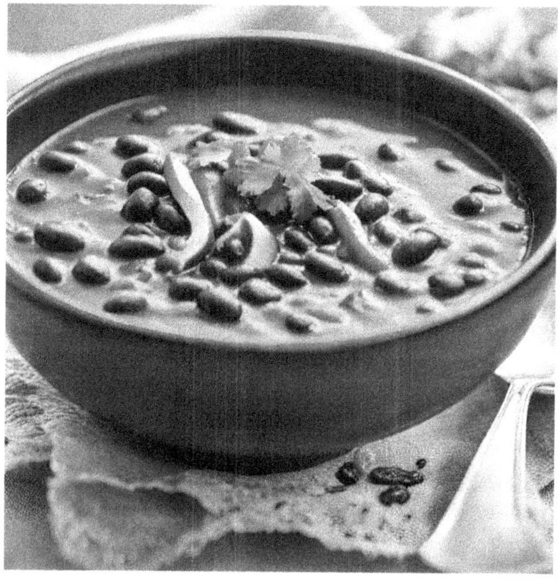

16. Beef Stew with Root Vegetables

Ingredients

- 1 lb beef stew meat, cubed
- 2 tablespoons olive oil
- 1 onion, chopped
- 3 garlic cloves, minced
- 2 carrots, chopped
- 2 parsnips, chopped
- 1 sweet potato, peeled and chopped
- 4 cups low-sodium beef broth
- 1 cup water
- 1 tablespoon tomato paste
- 1 teaspoon dried thyme
- 1 teaspoon dried rosemary
- 1 bay leaf

Instructions

1. In a large pot, heat the olive oil over medium heat. Add the beef and cook until browned on all sides, about 5 minutes.
2. Add the onion and garlic, and cook until softened, about 5 minutes.
3. Stir in the carrots, parsnips, sweet potato, beef broth, water, tomato paste, thyme, rosemary, and bay leaf.
4. Bring to a boil, then reduce the heat and simmer for 1.5 to 2 hours, or until the beef and vegetables are tender.
5. Remove the bay leaf.
6. Serve warm.

Nutrition Info (Per Serving)

- Calories: 350
- Protein: 30g
- Carbohydrates: 25g
- Fiber: 6g
- Sugars: 8g
- Fat: 15g

Servings: 4
Cooking Time: 2 hours

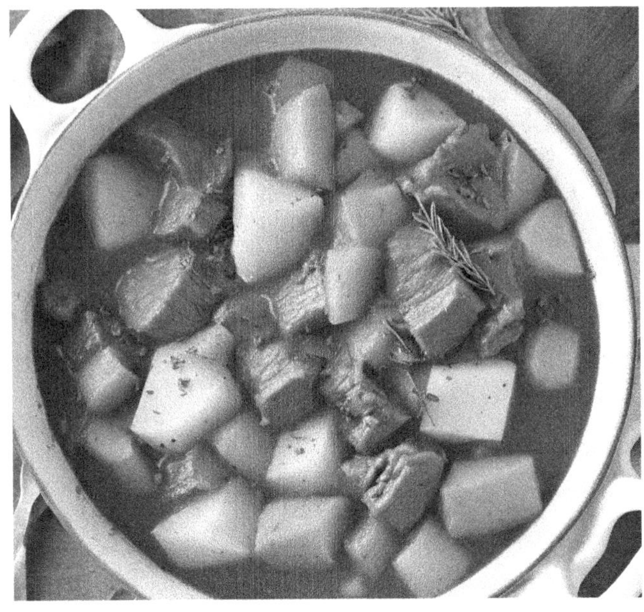

17. Squash and Pear Soup

Ingredients

- 2 tablespoons olive oil
- 1 onion, chopped
- 3 garlic cloves, minced
- 4 cups butternut squash, peeled and chopped
- 2 ripe pears, peeled, cored, and chopped
- 4 cups low-sodium vegetable broth
- 1/2 teaspoon ground cinnamon
- 1/4 teaspoon ground nutmeg
- 1/4 cup coconut milk
- 1 tablespoon fresh chives, chopped (for garnish)

Instructions

1. In a large pot, heat the olive oil over medium heat. Add the onion and garlic, and cook until softened, about 5 minutes.
2. Add the butternut squash, pears, vegetable broth, cinnamon, and nutmeg. Bring to a boil, then reduce the heat and simmer for 20-25 minutes, or until the squash and pears are tender.
3. Use an immersion blender to puree the soup until smooth, or transfer the soup to a blender and blend in batches.
4. Stir in the coconut milk and heat through.
5. Garnish with fresh chives.
6. Serve warm.

Nutrition Info (Per Serving)

- Calories: 180
- Protein: 2g
- Carbohydrates: 30g
- Fiber: 6g
- Sugars: 12g
- Fat: 7g

Servings: 4
Cooking Time: 30 minutes

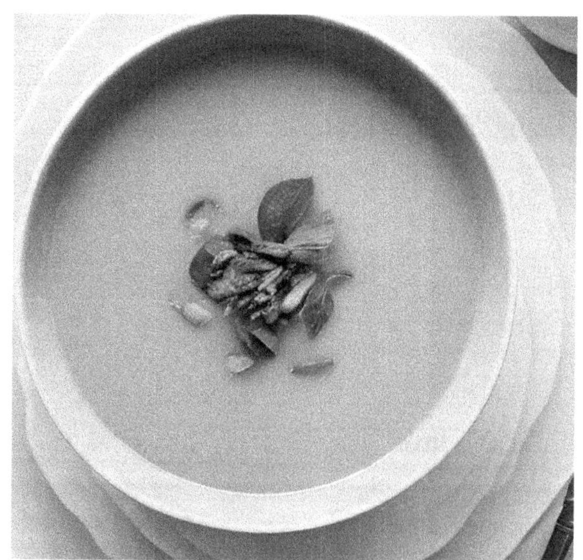

18. Cucumber and Avocado Gazpacho

Ingredients

- 2 large cucumbers, peeled and chopped
- 2 ripe avocados, peeled and pitted
- 1 green bell pepper, chopped
- 1/2 small red onion, chopped
- 2 garlic cloves, minced
- 1/4 cup fresh cilantro, chopped
- 2 tablespoons olive oil
- 2 tablespoons lime juice
- 2 cups cold water
- 1 teaspoon ground cumin

Instructions

1. In a blender, combine the cucumbers, avocados, green bell pepper, red onion, garlic, cilantro, olive oil, lime juice, cold water, and ground cumin.
2. Blend until smooth and creamy.
3. Chill the gazpacho in the refrigerator for at least 1 hour before serving.
4. Serve cold.

Nutrition Info (Per Serving)

- Calories: 180
- Protein: 3g
- Carbohydrates: 14g
- Fiber: 8g
- Sugars: 4g
- Fat: 14g

Servings: 4
Cooking Time: 10 minutes (plus 1 hour chilling)

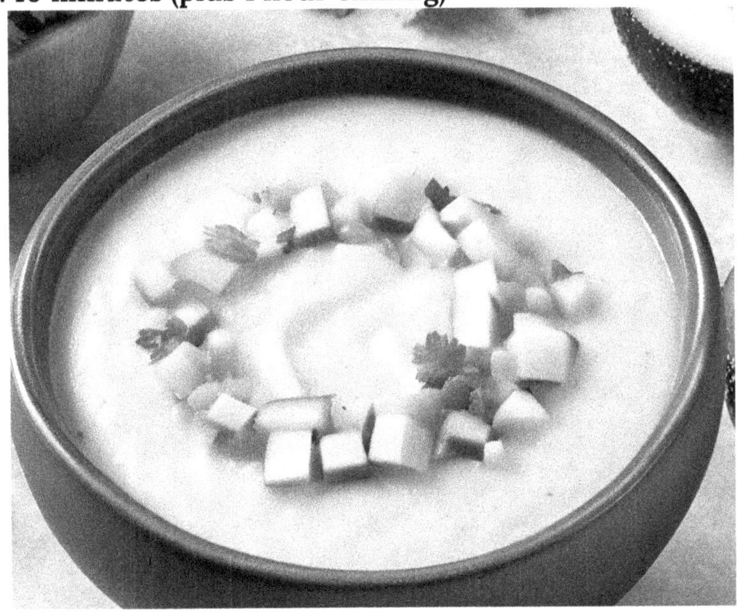

19. Cod and Corn Chowder

Ingredients

- 1 lb cod fillets, cut into chunks
- 2 tablespoons olive oil
- 1 onion, chopped
- 3 garlic cloves, minced
- 2 cups corn kernels (fresh or frozen)
- 2 potatoes, peeled and diced
- 4 cups low-sodium vegetable broth
- 1 cup unsweetened almond milk
- 1 teaspoon dried thyme
- 1/4 cup fresh parsley, chopped

Instructions

1. In a large pot, heat the olive oil over medium heat. Add the onion and garlic, and cook until softened, about 5 minutes.
2. Add the corn, potatoes, vegetable broth, almond milk, and dried thyme. Bring to a boil, then reduce the heat and simmer for 20 minutes, or until the potatoes are tender.
3. Add the cod chunks and cook for another 5-7 minutes, until the fish is cooked through and flakes easily.
4. Stir in the fresh parsley.
5. Serve warm.

Nutrition Info (Per Serving)

- Calories: 250
- Protein: 22g
- Carbohydrates: 30g
- Fiber: 5g
- Sugars: 6g
- Fat: 8g

Servings: 4
Cooking Time: 30 minutes

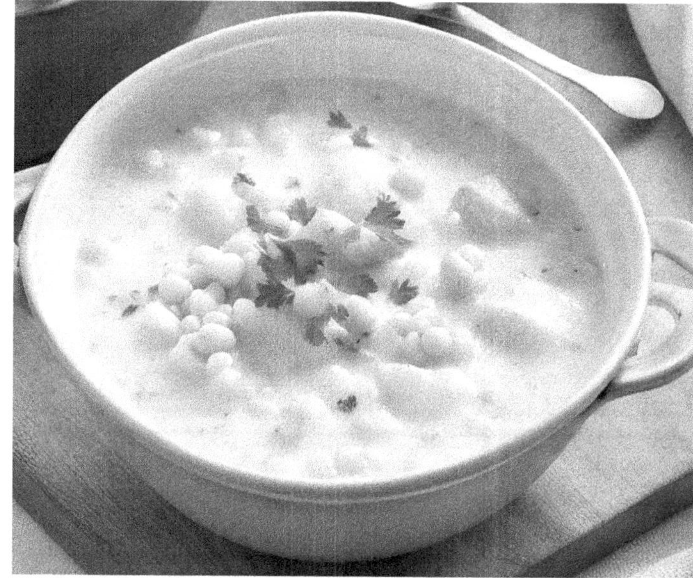

20. Chorizo and Kale Stew

Ingredients

- 1 lb chicken chorizo, sliced
- 2 tablespoons olive oil
- 1 onion, chopped
- 3 garlic cloves, minced
- 2 carrots, chopped
- 2 celery stalks, chopped
- 1 can (14.5 oz) diced tomatoes
- 4 cups low-sodium chicken broth
- 2 cups chopped kale
- 1 teaspoon smoked paprika
- 1/2 teaspoon ground cumin

Instructions

1. In a large pot, heat the olive oil over medium heat. Add the chorizo slices and cook until browned, about 5 minutes. Remove the chorizo and set aside.
2. In the same pot, add the onion, garlic, carrots, and celery. Cook until softened, about 5 minutes.
3. Stir in the diced tomatoes, chicken broth, smoked paprika, and cumin. Bring to a boil, then reduce the heat and simmer for 20 minutes.
4. Add the chopped kale and cooked chorizo. Simmer for another 10 minutes, until the kale is tender.
5. Serve warm.

Nutrition Info (Per Serving)

- Calories: 300
- Protein: 18g
- Carbohydrates: 20g
- Fiber: 6g
- Sugars: 7g
- Fat: 15g

Servings: 4
Cooking Time: 35 minutes

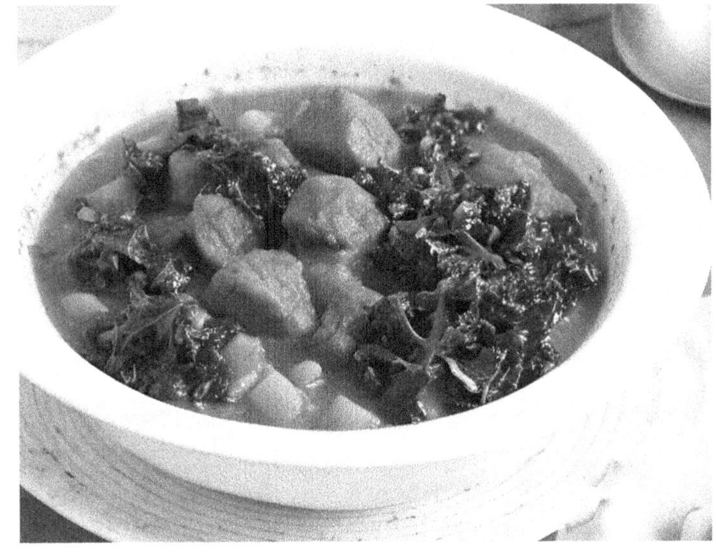

21. Mulligatawny Soup

Ingredients

- 2 tablespoons olive oil
- 1 onion, chopped
- 3 garlic cloves, minced
- 1 tablespoon grated fresh ginger
- 2 carrots, chopped
- 2 celery stalks, chopped
- 1 apple, peeled, cored, and chopped
- 1 tablespoon curry powder
- 1/2 teaspoon ground turmeric
- 1/4 teaspoon ground cinnamon
- 4 cups low-sodium chicken broth
- 1 cup coconut milk
- 1/2 cup red lentils, rinsed
- 1/4 cup fresh cilantro, chopped

Instructions

1. In a large pot, heat the olive oil over medium heat. Add the onion, garlic, ginger, carrots, celery, and apple. Cook until softened, about 5 minutes.
2. Stir in the curry powder, turmeric, and cinnamon, and cook for another minute.
3. Add the chicken broth, coconut milk, and red lentils. Bring to a boil, then reduce the heat and simmer for 20-25 minutes, or until the lentils are tender.
4. Use an immersion blender to puree the soup slightly, leaving some chunks for texture, or transfer half of the soup to a blender and blend until smooth, then return to the pot.
5. Garnish with fresh cilantro.
6. Serve warm.

Nutrition Info (Per Serving)

- Calories: 250
- Protein: 7g
- Carbohydrates: 30g
- Fiber: 8g
- Sugars: 10g
- Fat: 12g

Servings: 4
Cooking Time: 30 minutes

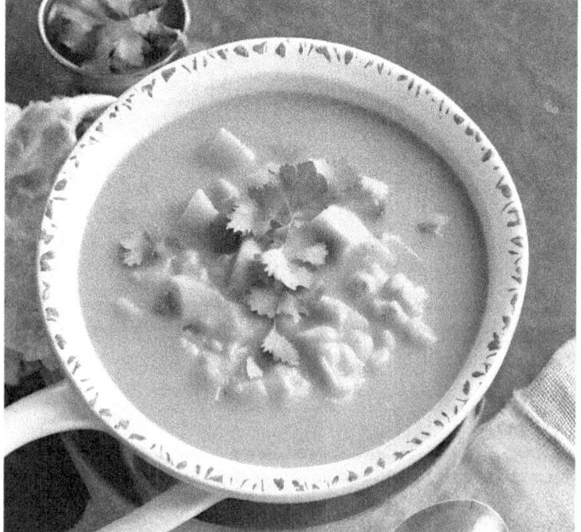

22. Szechuan Chicken Noodle Soup

Ingredients

- 1 lb boneless, skinless chicken breasts, thinly sliced
- 2 tablespoons olive oil
- 1 onion, chopped
- 3 garlic cloves, minced
- 1 tablespoon grated fresh ginger
- 1 red bell pepper, chopped
- 4 cups low-sodium chicken broth
- 1 cup water
- 2 tablespoons soy sauce or tamari
- 1 tablespoon rice vinegar
- 1 teaspoon Szechuan peppercorns, crushed
- 4 oz rice noodles
- 2 cups bok choy, chopped
- 1/4 cup fresh cilantro, chopped

Instructions

1. In a large pot, heat the olive oil over medium heat. Add the onion, garlic, ginger, and red bell pepper. Cook until softened, about 5 minutes.
2. Add the chicken slices and cook until no longer pink, about 5 minutes.
3. Stir in the chicken broth, water, soy sauce, rice vinegar, and crushed Szechuan peppercorns. Bring to a boil, then reduce the heat and simmer for 10 minutes.
4. Add the rice noodles and bok choy. Cook for another 5 minutes, until the noodles are tender.
5. Garnish with fresh cilantro.
6. Serve warm.

Nutrition Info (Per Serving)

- Calories: 300
- Protein: 25g
- Carbohydrates: 30g
- Fiber: 4g
- Sugars: 4g
- Fat: 10g

Servings: 4
Cooking Time: 30 minutes

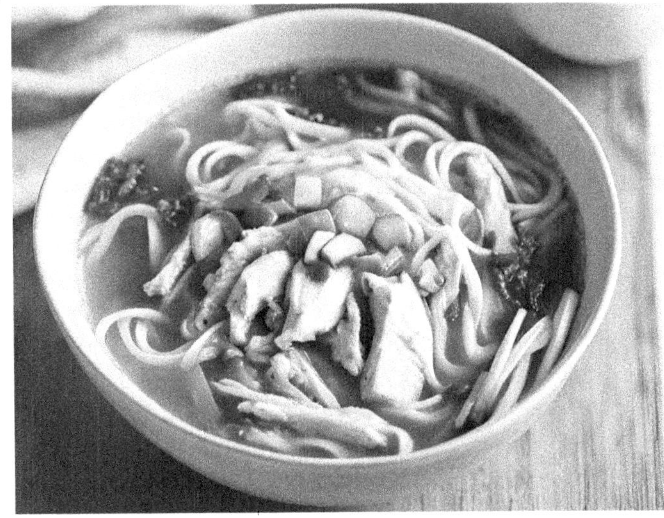

23. Zucchini Basil Soup

Ingredients

- 2 tablespoons olive oil
- 1 onion, chopped
- 3 garlic cloves, minced
- 4 cups chopped zucchini
- 4 cups low-sodium vegetable broth
- 1/2 cup fresh basil leaves
- 1/2 cup unsweetened almond milk
- 1/4 teaspoon ground nutmeg

Instructions

1. In a large pot, heat the olive oil over medium heat. Add the onion and garlic, and cook until softened, about 5 minutes.
2. Add the chopped zucchini and cook for another 5 minutes.
3. Stir in the vegetable broth and bring to a boil. Reduce the heat and simmer for 15 minutes, or until the zucchini is tender.
4. Use an immersion blender to puree the soup until smooth, or transfer the soup to a blender and blend in batches.
5. Stir in the basil leaves, almond milk, and nutmeg. Heat through.
6. Serve warm.

Nutrition Info (Per Serving)

- Calories: 150
- Protein: 3g
- Carbohydrates: 12g
- Fiber: 3g
- Sugars: 6g
- Fat: 10g

Servings: 4

Cooking Time: 25 minutes

Dessert and Snacks Recipes

1. Peach and Ginger Sorbet

Ingredients

- 4 cups frozen peaches
- 1 tablespoon fresh ginger, grated
- 1/4 cup honey
- 1/4 cup water
- Juice of 1 lemon

Instructions

1. In a blender or food processor, combine the frozen peaches, grated ginger, honey, water, and lemon juice.
2. Blend until smooth and creamy.
3. Transfer the mixture to a freezer-safe container and freeze for at least 2 hours, or until firm.
4. Serve cold.

Nutrition Info (Per Serving)

- Calories: 90
- Protein: 1g
- Carbohydrates: 22g
- Fiber: 2g
- Sugars: 18g
- Fat: 0g

Servings: 4

Cooking Time: 10 minutes (plus 2 hours freezing)

2. Dark Chocolate and Nut Bark

Ingredients

- 8 oz dark chocolate (70% cocoa or higher), chopped
- 1/4 cup almonds, chopped
- 1/4 cup walnuts, chopped
- 1/4 cup dried cranberries

Instructions

1. Line a baking sheet with parchment paper.
2. Melt the dark chocolate in a double boiler or microwave, stirring until smooth.
3. Stir in the chopped almonds, walnuts, and dried cranberries.
4. Pour the mixture onto the prepared baking sheet and spread evenly.
5. Refrigerate for at least 1 hour, or until the chocolate is firm.
6. Break into pieces and serve.

Nutrition Info (Per Serving)

- Calories: 180
- Protein: 3g
- Carbohydrates: 18g
- Fiber: 4g
- Sugars: 12g
- Fat: 12g

Servings: 8
Cooking Time: 10 minutes (plus 1 hour chilling)

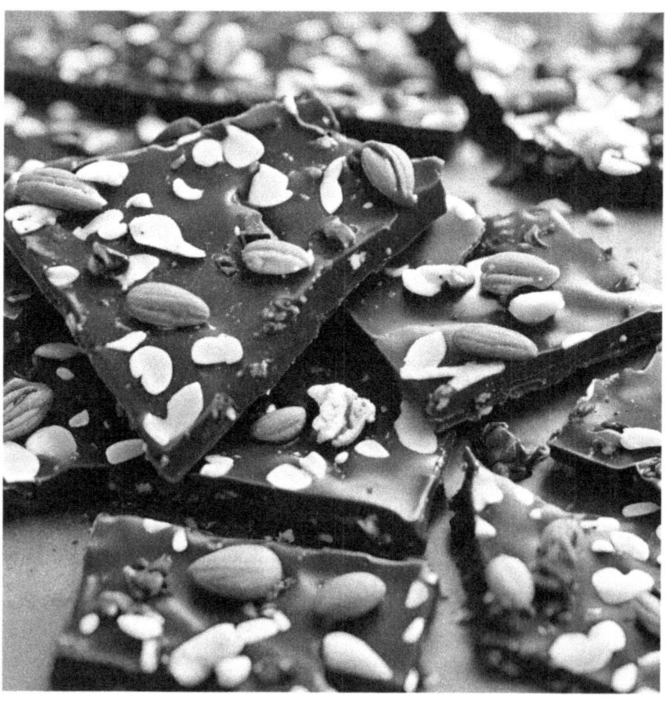

3. Oatmeal Raisin Cookies

Ingredients

- 1 cup gluten-free rolled oats
- 1/2 cup almond flour
- 1/4 cup coconut oil, melted
- 1/4 cup honey
- 1 egg
- 1/2 teaspoon baking soda
- 1 teaspoon ground cinnamon
- 1/2 cup raisins

Instructions

1. Preheat the oven to 350°F (175°C) and line a baking sheet with parchment paper.
2. In a large bowl, combine the rolled oats, almond flour, baking soda, and cinnamon.
3. In a separate bowl, whisk together the melted coconut oil, honey, and egg.
4. Add the wet ingredients to the dry ingredients and mix until well combined.
5. Fold in the raisins.
6. Drop spoonfuls of the dough onto the prepared baking sheet.
7. Bake for 10-12 minutes, or until the edges are golden brown.
8. Let cool before serving.

Nutrition Info (Per Serving)

- Calories: 120
- Protein: 2g
- Carbohydrates: 16g
- Fiber: 2g
- Sugars: 10g
- Fat: 6g

Servings: 12 cookies
Cooking Time: 15 minutes

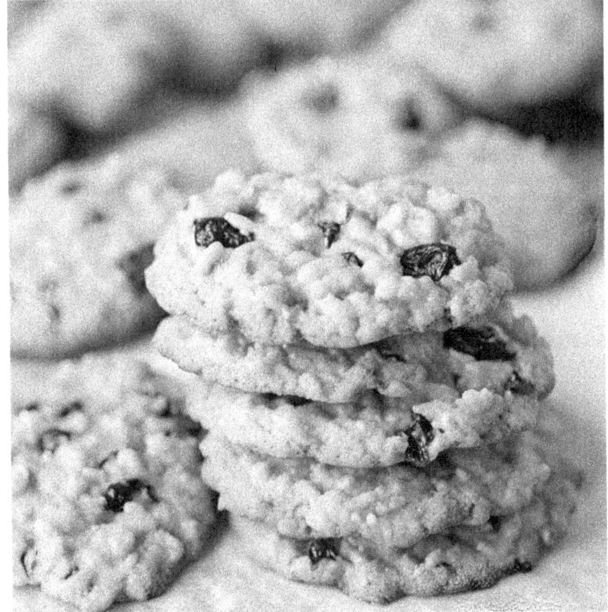

4. Pumpkin Spice Bread

Ingredients

- 1 1/2 cups almond flour
- 1/2 cup coconut flour
- 1 cup pumpkin puree
- 1/4 cup coconut oil, melted
- 1/4 cup honey
- 3 eggs
- 1 teaspoon baking soda
- 1 teaspoon ground cinnamon
- 1/2 teaspoon ground nutmeg
- 1/4 teaspoon ground cloves

Instructions

1. Preheat the oven to 350°F (175°C) and grease a loaf pan with coconut oil.
2. In a large bowl, whisk together the almond flour, coconut flour, baking soda, cinnamon, nutmeg, and cloves.
3. In another bowl, mix the pumpkin puree, melted coconut oil, honey, and eggs until smooth.
4. Add the wet ingredients to the dry ingredients and mix until well combined.
5. Pour the batter into the prepared loaf pan and smooth the top.
6. Bake for 45-50 minutes, or until a toothpick inserted into the center comes out clean.
7. Let cool before slicing and serving.

Nutrition Info (Per Serving)

- Calories: 180
- Protein: 5g
- Carbohydrates: 14g
- Fiber: 4g
- Sugars: 9g
- Fat: 12g

Servings: 10 slices

Cooking Time: 50 minutes

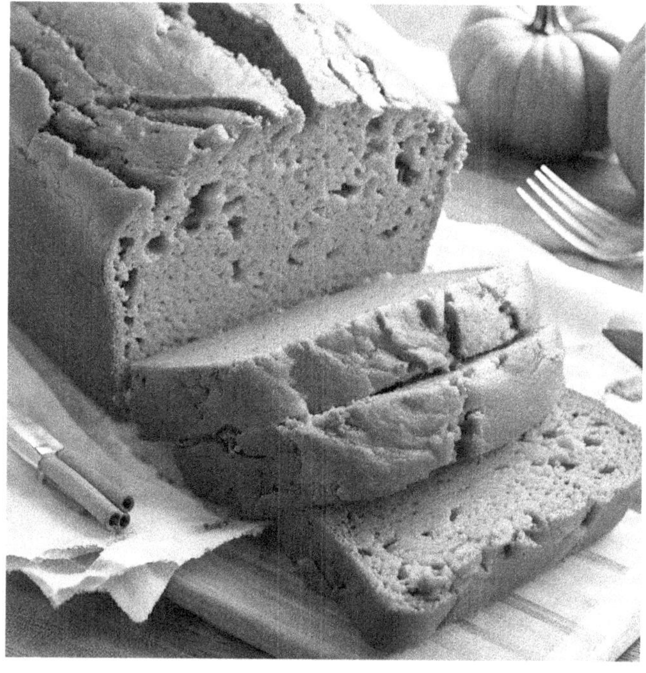

5. Lemon and Lavender Yogurt Cake

Ingredients

- 1 1/2 cups almond flour
- 1/2 cup coconut flour
- 1 cup Greek yogurt
- 1/4 cup coconut oil, melted
- 1/4 cup honey
- 3 eggs
- 1 teaspoon baking powder
- 1 teaspoon dried lavender
- Zest of 1 lemon
- Juice of 1 lemon

Instructions

1. Preheat the oven to 350°F (175°C) and grease a cake pan with coconut oil.
2. In a large bowl, whisk together the almond flour, coconut flour, and baking powder.
3. In another bowl, mix the Greek yogurt, melted coconut oil, honey, eggs, lemon zest, and lemon juice until smooth.
4. Add the wet ingredients to the dry ingredients and mix until well combined.
5. Stir in the dried lavender.
6. Pour the batter into the prepared cake pan and smooth the top.
7. Bake for 30-35 minutes, or until a toothpick inserted into the center comes out clean.
8. Let cool before slicing and serving.

Nutrition Info (Per Serving)

- Calories: 200
- Protein: 6g
- Carbohydrates: 18g
- Fiber: 4g
- Sugars: 10g
- Fat: 12g

Servings: 8

Cooking Time: 35 minutes

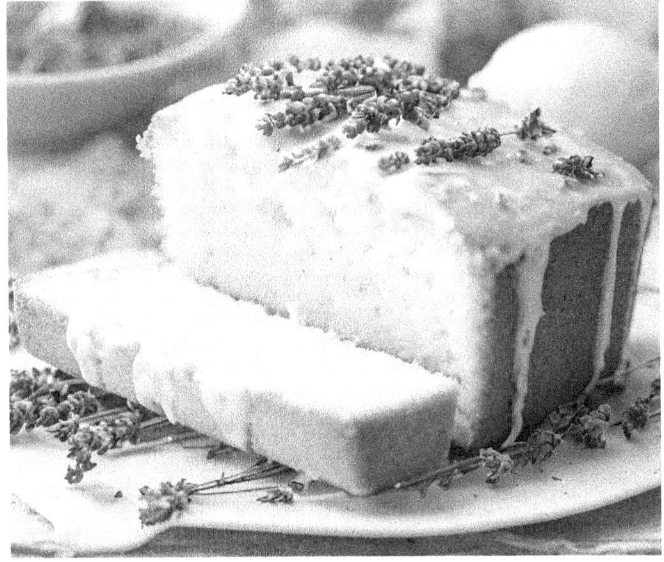

6. Banana and Oat Blender Pancakes

Ingredients

- 2 ripe bananas
- 2 eggs
- 1/2 cup gluten-free rolled oats
- 1/2 teaspoon baking powder
- 1 teaspoon vanilla extract
- 1/2 teaspoon ground cinnamon
- 1 tablespoon coconut oil (for cooking)

Instructions

1. In a blender, combine the bananas, eggs, rolled oats, baking powder, vanilla extract, and ground cinnamon. Blend until smooth.
2. Heat the coconut oil in a large skillet over medium heat.
3. Pour small circles of batter onto the skillet and cook for 2-3 minutes on each side, until golden brown and cooked through.
4. Serve warm.

Nutrition Info (Per Serving)

- Calories: 120
- Protein: 4g
- Carbohydrates: 18g
- Fiber: 3g
- Sugars: 7g
- Fat: 4g

Servings: 8 pancakes
Cooking Time: 15 minutes

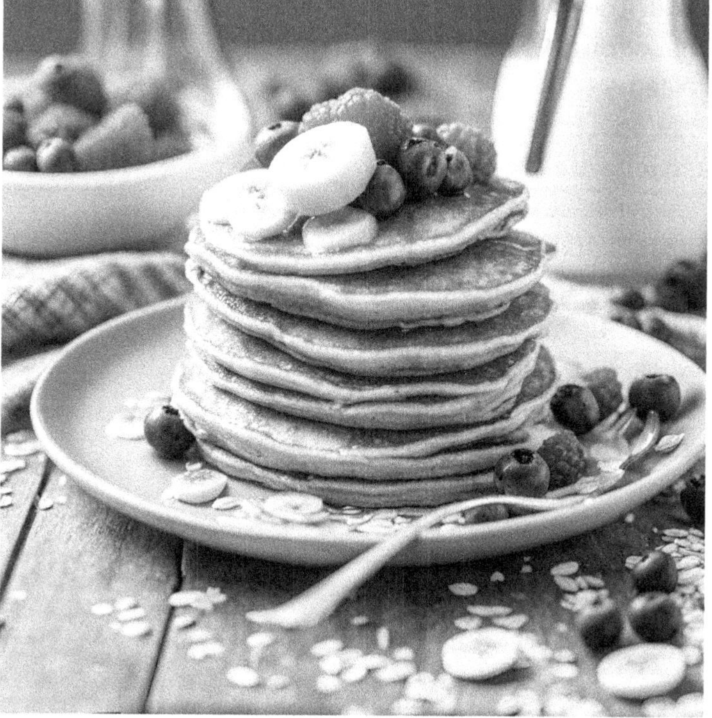

7. Hummus with Sliced Cucumbers

Ingredients

- 1 can (15 oz) chickpeas, drained and rinsed
- 1/4 cup tahini
- 2 tablespoons olive oil
- 2 tablespoons lemon juice
- 2 garlic cloves, minced
- 1 teaspoon ground cumin
- 1/4 cup water
- 2 cucumbers, sliced

Instructions

1. In a food processor, combine the chickpeas, tahini, olive oil, lemon juice, garlic, cumin, and water.
2. Blend until smooth and creamy, adding more water if needed to reach the desired consistency.
3. Serve the hummus with sliced cucumbers.

Nutrition Info (Per Serving)

- Calories: 120
- Protein: 3g
- Carbohydrates: 10g
- Fiber: 3g
- Sugars: 1g
- Fat: 8g

Servings: 4
Cooking Time: 10 minutes

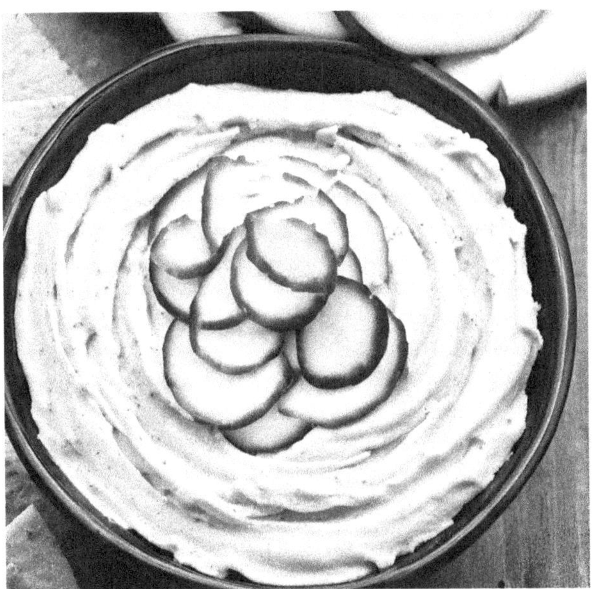

10-WEEK MEAL PLAN

Week 1

Day 1

- Breakfast: Chia Seed Pudding with Berries
- Lunch: Grilled Chicken with Avocado Salsa
- Snack: Hummus with Sliced Cucumbers
- Dinner: Turmeric Lentil Stew

Day 2

- Breakfast: Turmeric and Ginger Oatmeal
- Lunch: Shrimp and Avocado Salad
- Snack: Roasted Chickpeas
- Dinner: Baked Haddock with Tomato and Basil

Day 3

- Breakfast: Smoothie Bowl with Spinach and Avocado
- Lunch: Chicken and Spinach Stuffed Sweet Peppers
- Snack: Stuffed Dates with Almond Paste
- Dinner: Sweet Potato and Roasted Red Pepper Soup

Day 4

- Breakfast: Gluten-Free Banana Pancakes
- Lunch: Thai Coconut Shrimp Soup
- Snack: Dark Chocolate and Nut Bark
- Dinner: Chicken Quinoa Salad with Olive Oil Dressing

Day 5

- Breakfast: Buckwheat Porridge with Honey and Walnuts
- Lunch: Italian Lentil Soup
- Snack: Edamame Beans
- Dinner: Grilled Salmon with Dill and Lemon

Day 6

- Breakfast: Baked Sweet Potato with Greek Yogurt
- Lunch: Mushroom and Barley Soup
- Snack: Banana and Oat Blender Pancakes
- Dinner: Cod and Corn Chowder

Day 7

- Breakfast: Savory Muffins with Zucchini and Carrot
- Lunch: Chicken Salad with Walnuts and Dried Cranberries
- Snack: Peach and Ginger Sorbet
- Dinner: Beef Stew with Root Vegetables

Week 2

Day 1
- Breakfast: Smoked Salmon and Avocado Toast on Gluten-Free Bread
- Lunch: Spicy Black Bean Soup
- Snack: Oatmeal Raisin Cookies
- Dinner: Moroccan Spiced Chickpea Soup

Day 2
- Breakfast: Almond Butter and Banana Smoothie
- Lunch: Roasted Chicken with Root Vegetables
- Snack: Pumpkin Spice Bread
- Dinner: Miso Soup with Tofu and Seaweed

Day 3
- Breakfast: Quinoa Salad with Cherry Tomatoes and Kale
- Lunch: Chicken Bone Broth
- Snack: Lemon and Lavender Yogurt Cake
- Dinner: Grilled Trout with Parsley Salad

Day 4
- Breakfast: Stewed Pears with Cinnamon and Clove
- Lunch: Seafood Paella with Brown Rice
- Snack: Hummus with Sliced Cucumbers
- Dinner: Chorizo and Kale Stew

Day 5
- Breakfast: Kale and Blueberry Smoothie
- Lunch: Zucchini Basil Soup
- Snack: Roasted Chickpeas
- Dinner: Chicken and Barley Soup

Day 6
- Breakfast: Gluten-Free Apple Muffins
- Lunch: Poached Chicken Breast with Ginger Soy Sauce
- Snack: Dark Chocolate and Nut Bark
- Dinner: Chicken Piccata with Capers

Day 7
- Breakfast: Greek Yogurt Parfait with Mixed Nuts and Honey
- Lunch: Squash and Pear Soup
- Snack: Banana and Oat Blender Pancakes
- Dinner: Szechuan Chicken Noodle Soup

Week 3

Day 1
- Breakfast: Ricotta and Basil Omelet
- Lunch: Kale and White Bean Soup
- Snack: Peach and Ginger Sorbet
- Dinner: Clam Chowder with Sweet Potatoes

Day 2
- Breakfast: Pumpkin Seed Granola with Almond Milk
- Lunch: Grilled Chicken with Avocado Salsa
- Snack: Stuffed Dates with Almond Paste
- Dinner: Chicken and Vegetable Kabobs

Day 3
- Breakfast: Avocado and Egg Breakfast Pizza on Cauliflower Crust
- Lunch: Italian Lentil Soup
- Snack: Oatmeal Raisin Cookies
- Dinner: Lemon Garlic Butter Shrimp

Day 4
- Breakfast: Berry and Yogurt Smoothie
- Lunch: Chicken and Spinach Stuffed Sweet Peppers
- Snack: Edamame Beans
- Dinner: Spicy Grilled Mackerel

Day 5
- Breakfast: Sweet Potato and Black Bean Breakfast Burrito
- Lunch: Split Pea Soup with Ham
- Snack: Pumpkin Spice Bread
- Dinner: Chicken Bone Broth

Day 6
- Breakfast: Millet Porridge with Apples and Nuts
- Lunch: Chicken Gumbo with Okra
- Snack: Lemon and Lavender Yogurt Cake
- Dinner: Mushroom and Barley Soup

Day 7
- Breakfast: Cucumber and Hummus on Rice Cakes
- Lunch: Tomato Basil Soup
- Snack: Hummus with Sliced Cucumbers
- Dinner: Cedar Plank Salmon with Rosemary

Week 4

Day 1
- Breakfast: Coconut Yogurt with Mango and Flaxseed
- Lunch: Thai Coconut Shrimp Soup
- Snack: Roasted Chickpeas
- Dinner: Chicken Quinoa Salad with Olive Oil Dressing

Day 2
- Breakfast: Oat Bran Muffins with Prunes
- Lunch: Beetroot and Ginger Soup
- Snack: Dark Chocolate and Nut Bark
- Dinner: Grilled Salmon with Dill and Lemon

Day 3
- Breakfast: Gluten-Free Blueberry Waffles
- Lunch: Chicken and Barley Soup
- Snack: Peach and Ginger Sorbet
- Dinner: Cod and Corn Chowder

Day 4
- Breakfast: Kefir with Mixed Berries
- Lunch: Mulligatawny Soup
- Snack: Banana and Oat Blender Pancakes
- Dinner: Clam Chowder with Sweet Potatoes

Day 5
- Breakfast: Chia Seed Pudding with Berries
- Lunch: Mushroom and Barley Soup
- Snack: Stuffed Dates with Almond Paste
- Dinner: Moroccan Spiced Chickpea Soup

Day 6
- Breakfast: Turmeric and Ginger Oatmeal
- Lunch: Seafood Paella with Brown Rice
- Snack: Oatmeal Raisin Cookies
- Dinner: Chicken and Spinach Stuffed Sweet Peppers

Day 7
- Breakfast: Smoothie Bowl with Spinach and Avocado
- Lunch: Tomato Basil Soup
- Snack: Edamame Beans
- Dinner: Spicy Black Bean Soup

Week 5

Day 1
- Breakfast: Gluten-Free Banana Pancakes
- Lunch: Kale and White Bean Soup
- Snack: Dark Chocolate and Nut Bark
- Dinner: Sweet Potato and Roasted Red Pepper Soup

Day 2
- Breakfast: Buckwheat Porridge with Honey and Walnuts
- Lunch: Chicken Salad with Walnuts and Dried Cranberries
- Snack: Pumpkin Spice Bread
- Dinner: Chicken Piccata with Capers

Day 3
- Breakfast: Baked Sweet Potato with Greek Yogurt
- Lunch: Squash and Pear Soup
- Snack: Lemon and Lavender Yogurt Cake
- Dinner: Mushroom and Barley Soup

Day 4
- Breakfast: Savory Muffins with Zucchini and Carrot
- Lunch: Spicy Grilled Mackerel
- Snack: Hummus with Sliced Cucumbers
- Dinner: Chicken and Vegetable Kabobs

Day 5
- Breakfast: Smoked Salmon and Avocado Toast on Gluten-Free Bread
- Lunch: Moroccan Spiced Chickpea Soup
- Snack: Edamame Beans
- Dinner: Cedar Plank Salmon with Rosemary

Day 6
- Breakfast: Almond Butter and Banana Smoothie
- Lunch: Szechuan Chicken Noodle Soup
- Snack: Banana and Oat Blender Pancakes
- Dinner: Chicken Gumbo with Okra

Day 7
- Breakfast: Quinoa Salad with Cherry Tomatoes and Kale
- Lunch: Clam Chowder with Sweet Potatoes
- Snack: Peach and Ginger Sorbet
- Dinner: Chicken Quinoa Salad with Olive Oil Dressing

Week 6

Day 1
- Breakfast: Avocado and Egg Breakfast Pizza on Cauliflower Crust
- Lunch: Chicken and Sweet Potato Stew
- Snack: Greek Yogurt Parfait with Mixed Nuts and Honey
- Dinner: Beetroot and Ginger Soup

Day 2
- Breakfast: Buckwheat Porridge with Honey and Walnuts
- Lunch: Grilled Chicken with Avocado Salsa
- Snack: Dark Chocolate and Nut Bark
- Dinner: Baked Haddock with Tomato and Basil

Day 3
- Breakfast: Almond Butter and Banana Smoothie
- Lunch: Zucchini Basil Soup
- Snack: Peach and Ginger Sorbet
- Dinner: Chicken and Vegetable Kabobs

Day 4
- Breakfast: Greek Yogurt Parfait with Mixed Nuts and Honey
- Lunch: Split Pea Soup with Ham
- Snack: Oatmeal Raisin Cookies
- Dinner: Clam Chowder with Sweet Potatoes

Day 5
- Breakfast: Pumpkin Seed Granola with Almond Milk
- Lunch: Spicy Black Bean Soup
- Snack: Roasted Chickpeas
- Dinner: Chicken Piccata with Capers

Day 6
- Breakfast: Stewed Pears with Cinnamon and Clove
- Lunch: Thai Coconut Shrimp Soup
- Snack: Stuffed Dates with Almond Paste
- Dinner: Beef Stew with Root Vegetables

Day 7
- Breakfast: Oat Bran Muffins with Prunes
- Lunch: Mushroom and Barley Soup
- Snack: Hummus with Sliced Cucumbers
- Dinner: Lemon Garlic Butter Shrimp

Week 7

Day 1
- Breakfast: Ricotta and Basil Omelet
- Lunch: Chicken Salad with Walnuts and Dried Cranberries
- Snack: Dark Chocolate and Nut Bark
- Dinner: Chicken and Spinach Stuffed Sweet Peppers

Day 2
- Breakfast: Quinoa Salad with Cherry Tomatoes and Kale
- Lunch: Moroccan Spiced Chickpea Soup
- Snack: Greek Yogurt Parfait with Mixed Nuts and Honey
- Dinner: Cedar Plank Salmon with Rosemary

Day 3
- Breakfast: Kale and Blueberry Smoothie
- Lunch: Sweet Potato and Roasted Red Pepper Soup
- Snack: Oatmeal Raisin Cookies
- Dinner: Grilled Trout with Parsley Salad

Day 4
- Breakfast: Almond Butter and Banana Smoothie
- Lunch: Chicken Quinoa Salad with Olive Oil Dressing
- Snack: Roasted Chickpeas
- Dinner: Chicken Bone Broth

Day 5
- Breakfast: Pumpkin Seed Granola with Almond Milk
- Lunch: Clam Chowder with Sweet Potatoes
- Snack: Peach and Ginger Sorbet
- Dinner: Spicy Grilled Mackerel

Day 6
- Breakfast: Oat Bran Muffins with Prunes
- Lunch: Italian Lentil Soup
- Snack: Stuffed Dates with Almond Paste
- Dinner: Mushroom and Barley Soup

Day 7
- Breakfast: Stewed Pears with Cinnamon and Clove
- Lunch: Zucchini Basil Soup
- Snack: Hummus with Sliced Cucumbers
- Dinner: Chicken and Barley Soup

Week 8

Day 1
- Breakfast: Ricotta and Basil Omelet
- Lunch: Spicy Black Bean Soup
- Snack: Greek Yogurt Parfait with Mixed Nuts and Honey
- Dinner: Moroccan Spiced Chickpea Soup

Day 2
  * Breakfast: Greek Yogurt Parfait with Mixed Nuts and Honey
  * Lunch: Mushroom and Barley Soup
  * Snack: Oatmeal Raisin Cookies
  * Dinner: Baked Haddock with Tomato and Basil

Day 3
  * Breakfast: Kale and Blueberry Smoothie
  * Lunch: Chicken Piccata with Capers
  * Snack: Dark Chocolate and Nut Bark
  * Dinner: Lemon Garlic Butter Shrimp

Day 4
  * Breakfast: Pumpkin Seed Granola with Almond Milk
  * Lunch: Sweet Potato and Roasted Red Pepper Soup
  * Snack: Peach and Ginger Sorbet
  * Dinner: Chicken Quinoa Salad with Olive Oil Dressing

Day 5
  * Breakfast: Oat Bran Muffins with Prunes
  * Lunch: Split Pea Soup with Ham
  * Snack: Roasted Chickpeas
  * Dinner: Clam Chowder with Sweet Potatoes

Day 6
  * Breakfast: Stewed Pears with Cinnamon and Clove
  * Lunch: Zucchini Basil Soup
  * Snack: Stuffed Dates with Almond Paste
  * Dinner: Grilled Trout with Parsley Salad

Day 7
  * Breakfast: Ricotta and Basil Omelet
  * Lunch: Chicken and Spinach Stuffed Sweet Peppers
  * Snack: Greek Yogurt Parfait with Mixed Nuts and Honey
  * Dinner: Beef Stew with Root Vegetables

Week 9

Day 1
  * Breakfast: Kale and Blueberry Smoothie
  * Lunch: Mushroom and Barley Soup
  * Snack: Oatmeal Raisin Cookies
  * Dinner: Chicken and Barley Soup

Day 2
- Breakfast: Pumpkin Seed Granola with Almond Milk
- Lunch: Spicy Black Bean Soup
- Snack: Dark Chocolate and Nut Bark
- Dinner: Moroccan Spiced Chickpea Soup

Day 3
- Breakfast: Oat Bran Muffins with Prunes
- Lunch: Chicken Quinoa Salad with Olive Oil Dressing
- Snack: Peach and Ginger Sorbet
- Dinner: Baked Haddock with Tomato and Basil

Day 4
- Breakfast: Stewed Pears with Cinnamon and Clove
- Lunch: Zucchini Basil Soup
- Snack: Roasted Chickpeas
- Dinner: Lemon Garlic Butter Shrimp

Day 5
- Breakfast: Ricotta and Basil Omelet
- Lunch: Clam Chowder with Sweet Potatoes
- Snack: Greek Yogurt Parfait with Mixed Nuts and Honey
- Dinner: Chicken Piccata with Capers

Day 6
- Breakfast: Kale and Blueberry Smoothie
- Lunch: Sweet Potato and Roasted Red Pepper Soup
- Snack: Stuffed Dates with Almond Paste
- Dinner: Grilled Trout with Parsley Salad

Day 7
- Breakfast: Pumpkin Seed Granola with Almond Milk
- Lunch: Split Pea Soup with Ham
- Snack: Oatmeal Raisin Cookies
- Dinner: Chicken Quinoa Salad with Olive Oil Dressing

Week 10

Day 1
- Breakfast: Oat Bran Muffins with Prunes
- Lunch: Moroccan Spiced Chickpea Soup
- Snack: Greek Yogurt Parfait with Mixed Nuts and Honey
- Dinner: Chicken and Spinach Stuffed Sweet Peppers

Day 2
- Breakfast: Stewed Pears with Cinnamon and Clove
- Lunch: Mushroom and Barley Soup
- Snack: Dark Chocolate and Nut Bark
- Dinner: Spicy Black Bean Soup

Day 3
- Breakfast: Ricotta and Basil Omelet
- Lunch: Zucchini Basil Soup
- Snack: Peach and Ginger Sorbet
- Dinner: Baked Haddock with Tomato and Basil

Day 4
- Breakfast: Kale and Blueberry Smoothie
- Lunch: Chicken Piccata with Capers
- Snack: Roasted Chickpeas
- Dinner: Clam Chowder with Sweet Potatoes

Day 5
- Breakfast: Pumpkin Seed Granola with Almond Milk
- Lunch: Chicken Quinoa Salad with Olive Oil Dressing
- Snack: Oatmeal Raisin Cookies
- Dinner: Lemon Garlic Butter Shrimp

Day 6
- Breakfast: Oat Bran Muffins with Prunes
- Lunch: Sweet Potato and Roasted Red Pepper Soup
- Snack: Stuffed Dates with Almond Paste
- Dinner: Grilled Trout with Parsley Salad

Day 7
- Breakfast: Stewed Pears with Cinnamon and Clove
- Lunch: Spicy Black Bean Soup
- Snack: Greek Yogurt Parfait with Mixed Nuts and Honey
- Dinner: Chicken and Barley Soup

WEEKLY MEAL PLANNER + WORKBOOK

	BREAKFAST	LUNCH	DINNER	SNACKS
MONDAY				
TUESDAY				
WEDNESDAY				
THURSDAY				
FRIDAY				
SATURDAY				
SUNDAY				

What are your current dietary habits, and how do you think they impact your rheumatoid arthritis symptoms?

WEEKLY MEAL PLANNER + WORKBOOK

	BREAKFAST	LUNCH	DINNER	SNACKS
MONDAY				
TUESDAY				
WEDNESDAY				
THURSDAY				
FRIDAY				
SATURDAY				
SUNDAY				

How often do you experience flare-ups, and what foods do you suspect might be contributing to them?

....

....

....

....

....

....

WEEKLY MEAL PLANNER + WORKBOOK

	BREAKFAST	LUNCH	DINNER	SNACKS
MONDAY				
TUESDAY				
WEDNESDAY				
THURSDAY				
FRIDAY				
SATURDAY				
SUNDAY				

Which anti-inflammatory foods are you most excited to incorporate into your diet, and why?

WEEKLY MEAL PLANNER + WORKBOOK

	BREAKFAST	LUNCH	DINNER	SNACKS
MONDAY				
TUESDAY				
WEDNESDAY				
THURSDAY				
FRIDAY				
SATURDAY				
SUNDAY				

List three goals you hope to achieve by following the rheumatoid arthritis diet. How will you measure your progress?

WEEKLY MEAL PLANNER + WORKBOOK

	BREAKFAST	LUNCH	DINNER	SNACKS
MONDAY				
TUESDAY				
WEDNESDAY				
THURSDAY				
FRIDAY				
SATURDAY				
SUNDAY				

What are some challenges you anticipate facing while transitioning to the rheumatoid arthritis diet, and how can you prepare to overcome them?

....

....

....

....

....

....

WEEKLY MEAL PLANNER + WORKBOOK

	BREAKFAST	LUNCH	DINNER	SNACKS
MONDAY				
TUESDAY				
WEDNESDAY				
THURSDAY				
FRIDAY				
SATURDAY				
SUNDAY				

How do you plan to track your meals and symptoms to identify any correlations between food and flare-ups?

WEEKLY MEAL PLANNER + WORKBOOK

	BREAKFAST	LUNCH	DINNER	SNACKS
MONDAY				
TUESDAY				
WEDNESDAY				
THURSDAY				
FRIDAY				
SATURDAY				
SUNDAY				

Are there any foods or ingredients you are concerned about eliminating from your diet? Why?

WEEKLY MEAL PLANNER + WORKBOOK

	BREAKFAST	LUNCH	DINNER	SNACKS
MONDAY				
TUESDAY				
WEDNESDAY				
THURSDAY				
FRIDAY				
SATURDAY				
SUNDAY				

How can you involve your family or friends in your dietary changes to make the transition easier and more enjoyable?

WEEKLY MEAL PLANNER + WORKBOOK

	BREAKFAST	LUNCH	DINNER	SNACKS
MONDAY				
TUESDAY				
WEDNESDAY				
THURSDAY				
FRIDAY				
SATURDAY				
SUNDAY				

What role do you think hydration plays in managing your rheumatoid arthritis symptoms, and how will you ensure you stay adequately hydrated?

WEEKLY MEAL PLANNER + WORKBOOK

	BREAKFAST	LUNCH	DINNER	SNACKS
MONDAY				
TUESDAY				
WEDNESDAY				
THURSDAY				
FRIDAY				
SATURDAY				
SUNDAY				

How will you handle social situations or dining out while following the rheumatoid arthritis diet?

WEEKLY MEAL PLANNER + WORKBOOK

	BREAKFAST	LUNCH	DINNER	SNACKS
MONDAY				
TUESDAY				
WEDNESDAY				
THURSDAY				
FRIDAY				
SATURDAY				
SUNDAY				

Which recipes from the meal plan are you most looking forward to trying, and why?

WEEKLY MEAL PLANNER + WORKBOOK

	BREAKFAST	LUNCH	DINNER	SNACKS
MONDAY				
TUESDAY				
WEDNESDAY				
THURSDAY				
FRIDAY				
SATURDAY				
SUNDAY				

What are some non-food-related strategies you can use to manage your rheumatoid arthritis symptoms alongside your new diet?

WEEKLY MEAL PLANNER + WORKBOOK

	BREAKFAST	LUNCH	DINNER	SNACKS
MONDAY				
TUESDAY				
WEDNESDAY				
THURSDAY				
FRIDAY				
SATURDAY				
SUNDAY				

What are some signs of improvement you will look for to gauge the effectiveness of the rheumatoid arthritis diet?

....

....

....

....

....

....

WEEKLY MEAL PLANNER + WORKBOOK

	BREAKFAST	LUNCH	DINNER	SNACKS
MONDAY				
TUESDAY				
WEDNESDAY				
THURSDAY				
FRIDAY				
SATURDAY				
SUNDAY				

How do you plan to handle any setbacks or challenges you encounter while following the rheumatoid arthritis diet?

Scan the QR code below to get a surprise bonus!